O9-AIE-267

JUST EAT

BARRY ESTABROOK

JUST EAT

One Reporter's Quest for a Weight-Loss Regimen that Works

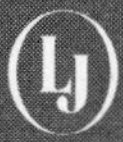

LORENA JONES BOOKS
An imprint of TEN SPEED PRESS
California | New York

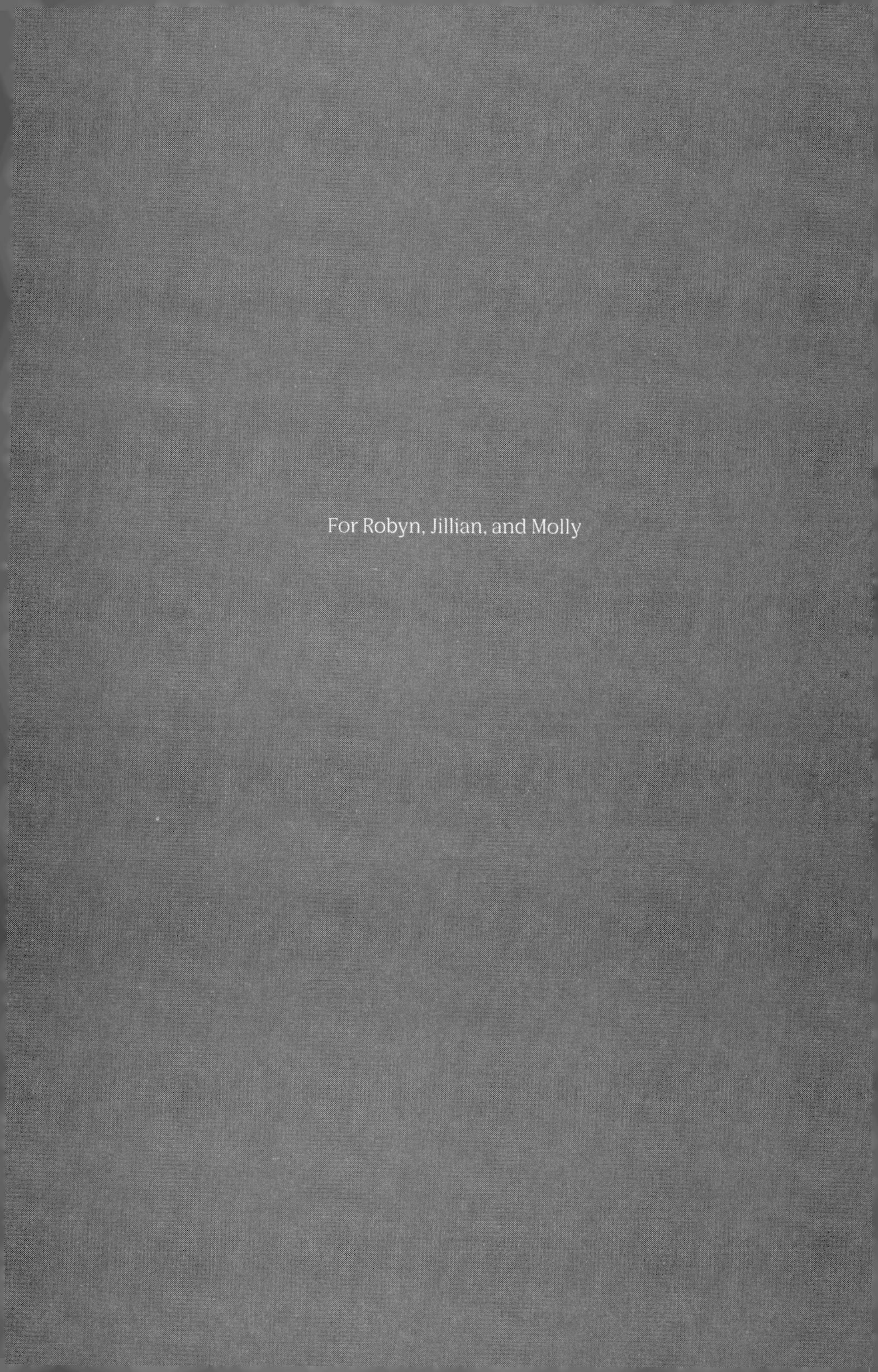

For Robyn, Jillian, and Molly

PROBABLY NOTHING
IN THE WORLD AROUSES
MORE FALSE HOPES THAN
THE FIRST FOUR HOURS
OF A DIET.

—SAMUEL BECKETT

CONTENTS

CHAPTER ONE

FORTY UNWANTED POUNDS—1

CHAPTER TWO

INSTANT RESULTS—15

CHAPTER THREE

DIET NATION—23

CHAPTER FOUR

THERE ARE ONLY THREE DIETS—35

CHAPTER FIVE

DEAN CUISINE—51

CHAPTER SIX

LOW-CARB COUNTRY—79

CHAPTER SEVEN

LOSERS PAY—101

CHAPTER EIGHT

HILL TRIBE—123

CHAPTER NINE

CLUB MED—135

CHAPTER TEN

A FRENCH CONNECTION—147

CHAPTER ELEVEN

THE RECKONING—159

CHAPTER TWELVE

BIG WINNERS—181

CHAPTER THIRTEEN

MINI ME—189

PRECURSORS TO LATE-TWENTIETH-CENTURY DIETS—198

NOTES—201 | BIBLIOGRAPHY—225

ACKNOWLEDGMENTS—235

INDEX—237

CHAPTER ONE

FORTY UNWANTED POUNDS

Dr. Dennis Beatty, my primary care physician for nearly two decades, has never been judgmental about my weight. He doesn't have to be. His very presence says everything that needs saying. Doctor Dennis, who is in his fifties, has a boyishly fair complexion and is as lean as a high-school track star. I am in my sixties, and no one would mistake my physique for that of an athletic teenager. I have spent many years as one of the seven in ten Americans whom the Centers for Disease Control and Prevention (CDC) says needs to lose weight—about forty pounds in my case.

At the end of a physical exam just before I marked a milestone birthday, I could tell from the discomforted look on Doctor Dennis's face that he was about to deliver news I did not want to hear. Rotating his laptop so that I could read the screen from where I perched in a hospital johnny on the examination table, he pointed to a series of numbers. My cholesterol was worryingly high, even though I had been taking medication to control it. In order to get it down, Doctor Dennis said he was going to up my dosage of atorvastatin to the maximum level he would prescribe. My blood pressure, he noted, was also elevated, despite a daily pill of irbesartan—again the maximum amount. Although he had run out of drug-based options, he told me there was one thing I could do to address both concerns.

I knew exactly what he was about to say. My wife, children, friends, and colleagues had all subtly suggested that I improve my eating and drinking habits to lose weight. Their advice inevitably came with an implied, if unspoken, "or else." My father had the first of his two heart attacks at fifty-eight and died of a stroke twelve years later. My brother died at age sixty-four of a sudden massive heart attack. One of my grandfathers developed type 2 diabetes during the last decades of his life. The other died prematurely from heart disease. I had no desire to continue that family tradition.

Those extra pounds had attached themselves to my belly insidiously over four decades, beginning shortly after I graduated from university. For most of that time, my weight never really bothered me. I was strong, physically active, and, as far as I could tell, my plumpness did not interfere with my professional, social, or romantic pursuits. But sitting there in Doctor Dennis's examination room, I realized that something had changed. My shirts strained against their buttons. The waistbands of my pants were uncomfortably tight. When walking down a street and catching sight of my reflection in shop windows, I recoiled. That lumpy character in no way fit the image I had of myself. I became embarrassed to take off my shirt at the beach. Hiking, cross-country skiing, and cycling—all activities I adore—were becoming less enjoyable as I huffed and puffed several yards behind my wife. There were still a lot of mountain trails I wanted to scramble over, lakes and rivers I hoped to paddle, and pools in which I planned to someday cast a fly. More wonderful than any mountain, an enchanting, impish granddaughter had entered my life, and I wanted to stick around to experience pleasures I had forgotten from when my daughters were growing up.

Joining the two-thirds of Americans who have medically significant amounts of weight to lose, I decided to go on a diet, something I'd never done. For the worst possible reason, I chose a regimen called the Whole30, yet I'll wager most people select their diets according to the same lame criteria: It happened to be the weight-loss fad du jour. There was no way to avoid hearing about it. *The Whole30: The 30-Day Guide to Total Health and Food Freedom*, the original book (there are now at least a half-dozen spinoffs) describing the diet's parameters and providing a hundred or so recipes, climbed to the top of the *New York Times* bestseller list, where it remained for more than a year. *Whole30* inspired a mini-industry overseen by Melissa Urban, one of the book's authors. In addition to sales of more than two million books, the company had millions of social media followers, made branding deals with the likes of Whole Foods Market and Blue Apron, the country's largest meal-delivery company. Segments featuring *Whole30's* youthful and oh-so-buff authors Urban and her then-husband Dallas Hartwig aired on *Today, Good Morning America, Nightline*, and many other national television programs. Publications, including *Cosmopolitan, Parade*, and the *Washington Post*, touted the diet's results. It seemed as if half the people my wife and I knew were "doing a Whole30" and had become "Whole30-ers," terms that Hartwig and Urban had coined.

The theory behind the Whole30 is that certain food groups damage our health, pack on pounds, and wreck the quality of our lives without our even realizing it. By eliminating "psychologically unhealthy, hormone-unbalancing, gut-disrupting, inflammatory food groups" for a full thirty days (hence the diet's name), I would cleanse my body and push the "reset" button on my health.

Like almost all creators of contemporary diets, Hartwig and Urban insist that theirs, unlike the others, is absolutely *not* a diet. Rather, they write, "It is self-experimentation to help you determine how the foods you've been eating are actually impacting you—your digestion, your metabolism, your immune system, your cravings, and your emotional relationship with food." They claim that it's an unintended consequence that 96 percent of the people who go on their diet—oops, I mean *self-experiment*—lose weight.

In practice, the Whole30 regimen is nothing short of draconian. Under Hartwig and Urban's mantra of "tough love," Whole30-ers are absolutely forbidden to consume dairy products. In Hartwig and Urban's world, milk, whether it comes from a cow, a goat, or a sheep, contains growth and immune factors (good for baby ungulates, bad for adult humans) and inflammatory proteins. It can provoke a high insulin response and has been associated with autoimmune diseases and cancers.

Whole30-ers must also "slay the Sugar Dragon" because added sugars from any source, including honey and maple syrup, provide empty calories that can lead to hormonal and metabolic problems and promote insulin resistance, diabetes, and obesity. Sugar substitutes are also verboten; they can disrupt gut bacteria, and they prevent you from conquering your sweet tooth. Alcohol of any type—even cooking wine—is banned because booze has the same ill effects as sugar, only worse, and is a neurotoxin to boot. Because they produce hormonal imbalance

THE Whole30 DIET

DO THIS

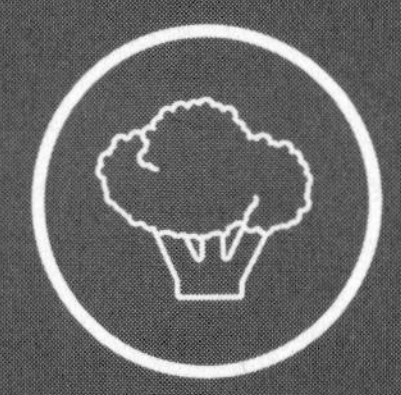

UNLIMITED MEAT,
ANIMAL FAT, FRUITS,
AND VEGETABLES

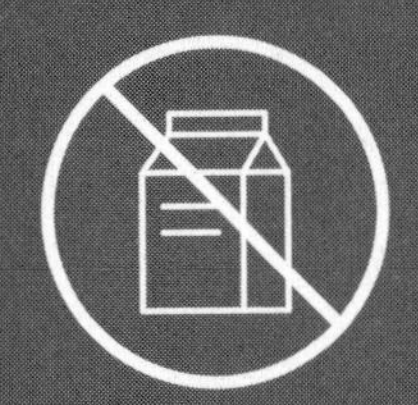

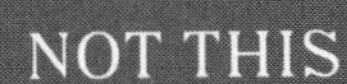

DAIRY

SUGAR

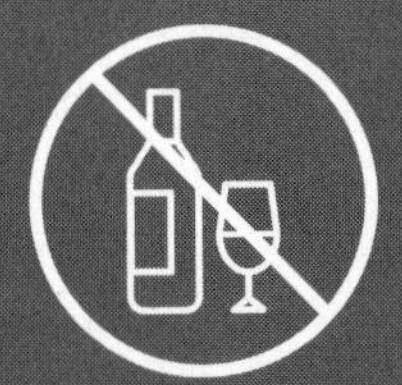

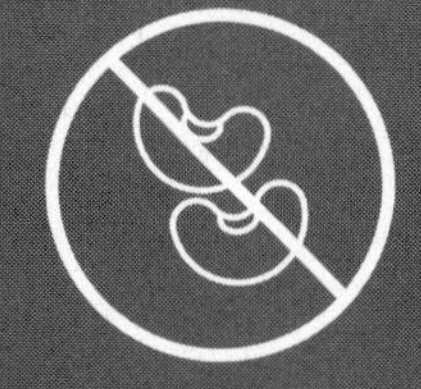

ALCOHOL

GRAINS OR
LEGUMES

and contain inflammatory proteins such as gluten, all grains, even whole grains, are banned. The Whole30 blacklist includes any foods that contain wheat, rice, corn, millet, or quinoa, a seed that was all the rage among conscientious eaters. Beans (including soy and soy products, like tofu) and peanuts must be avoided because they contain fermentable carbohydrates, which can cause an imbalance in gut bacteria.

Hartwig and Urban categorize everything we eat as either Whole30 Approved or not. There are no gray areas. Cheating or making even a small slip is strictly verboten. One tiny lapse—a sip of Pinot Noir, a nibble of cheddar, a dribble of skim milk in your coffee—even on the twenty-ninth day of a Whole30, requires going back to day one and starting all over again. Whole30-ers are also banned from weighing themselves for the duration of the program to prevent them from focusing on weight loss rather than enjoying all the other good things the diet is delivering.

But the rewards, Hartwig and Urban told Whole30-ers, would more than compensate for any short-term pain. Their book assured me that doing a Whole30 would change my life and leave me positively "glowing," a descriptor that no one to my knowledge had ever applied to me. My disposition would become "sunny," although I've been led to believe that it's often curmudgeonly. My veins would pulse with supercharged "tiger blood." I would enjoy effortless weight loss, better sleep, consistent energy, increased athletic performance, great sex, and other "miracles." In addition, my blood pressure would plummet, my cholesterol level would tumble, and any seasonal allergies would dry up.

Best of all, I would still be able to enjoy many of the foods that I like. Well-marbled rib steaks, for example. And the bright-yolked eggs my little flock of hens obligingly provide. Whole30-ers are encouraged to eat all the meat they want, including plenty of animal fat. Animal protein is included in every meal. Hartwig and Urban just asked that followers vary the types of meat they eat—if it's roast beef tonight, then it's pork chops or roast leg of lamb tomorrow. The list of Whole30 Approved fare also includes all kinds of poultry and seafood. The plan puts no limits on vegetables with the exception of chips and french fries.

I liked the idea that Whole30 had distinct beginning and end points, so I wouldn't have to confront the prospect of an infinite future devoid of cocktails or spoonfuls of ice cream. As a Whole30-er, I would have no obligation to measure portions and keep a running tally of daily calorie intake, which fit nicely with my aversion to having mathematical calculations and fitness apps come between me and what's for dinner. And after thirty days, I could start reintroducing the banned foodstuffs to my diet one at a time, being careful to monitor my body's reaction. If I reacted badly, that food group would have to be dropped permanently from my menu. If not, I could begin eating it again. The Whole30 was an experiment conducted by me, on me, to discover my ideal personalized diet.

Stripped of its catchy name and Hartwig and Urban's New Age–ish zeitgeist, the Whole30 is nothing more than another variation on the paleo diets that first became popular after an article by Dr. S. Boyd Eaton, an Atlanta radiologist, appeared in the *New England Journal of Medicine* in 1985. Eaton expanded upon the article in his book *The Paleolithic Prescription*. The assumption behind the paleo diet is that humans dramatically changed their eating habits about ten thousand years ago, when we abandoned nomadic hunter-gatherer living, established permanent settlements, and invented farming. We began eating and drinking items that we'd never consumed before, or had consumed in minuscule quantities. Those foods are precisely the ones Hartwig and Urban and other paleo advocates say we should avoid. They believe that a mere ten thousand years is far too short a period of time for our bodies to have evolved enough to accept these "new" foods. Our digestive systems, which developed over millions of years of hunting meat and gathering fruits and vegetables, are not equipped to deal with grains, legumes, sugar, milk, or alcohol. The paleo response to Michael Pollan's oft-quoted advice about not consuming anything your great-great-great grandmother wouldn't recognize as food is this: Don't eat anything your cave-dwelling, club-wielding Paleolithic ancestors wouldn't recognize as food.

But there is nothing old-fashioned about the key to the runaway success of Whole30. After its development in 2009, the Whole30 attracted little attention until 2014, when Hartwig and Urban cleverly tweaked the old paleo precepts to appeal to the social media set. Before embarking on a Whole30, participants are encouraged to invite friends, office mates, and family members to join them on the program. These groups support each other and exchange recipes on Twitter and Facebook. Followers swap images of their increasingly narrow waistlines on Instagram. They can join chat sessions, post suggestions, ask questions, or read the blog posts by Urban on the Whole30 website, and they can make new friends on the Whole30 forum and sign up for the Whole30 Daily, an electronic newsletter. *The Whole30* is the only diet book I've seen that includes a social media primer, which urges participants to get their hashtags in order and then explains exactly what a hashtag is and how to use #whole30 to make your Twitter and Facebook posts searchable. As friends shared their stories, and their followers saw the results and decided to try the diet themselves, the Whole30 went viral.

I decided to hop aboard the bandwagon. For one month, I would live "one bite at a time," as Hartwig and Urban say. What did I have to lose, aside from those extra pounds?

Plenty, it turned out.

Because I work from home, I had an innate advantage over most Whole30-ers: I didn't venture out daily into a minefield of muffins, pizzas, lattes, and after-work beers with office mates. Breakfasts were tolerable and filling but quickly became monotonous—there are only so many ways you can cook eggs without butter. Lunches were easy, thanks to my fondness for canned tuna, meaty leftovers from previous suppers, and fruit. Dinners at home never posed a problem. I could have my fill of chicken, beef, pork, lamb, and seafood. Thanks to the large garden that I tend, a cornucopia of fresh vegetables makes its way into our kitchen during the warm months. Yet, despite having no limit on the amount of Whole30 Approved foods that I could eat, I often felt half starved. Equally often, I felt stuffed and had to force myself to eat. To put it indelicately, constipation became an issue, as did its counterpart. Over the course of a month I was, by turns, grumpy, dull-witted, sleepy, dizzy, and plagued by cravings for all the wonderful things that had been outlawed from my plate and glass.

Halfway through my Whole30, I traveled to speak at a book festival in Decatur, an Atlanta suburb. In the airport, famished and waiting for my connecting flight, I could find nothing substantial that was Whole30 compliant, so I munched glumly on an overpriced packet of cashews. The first evening in town, I begged off going out to the popular Taqueria Del Sol with my wife and a fun-loving group of pals. I was that sad guy alone at the bar of a Ted's Montana Grill with a soda water and a bison patty topped by a few slices of raw onions and tasteless tomatoes—hold the bun, cheese, and condiments.

The real test of my willpower came the final night in Decatur, when I joined a group of food writers at Twain's Brewpub and Billiards, whose menu featured edgy twists on traditional Southern fare. Twain's chef at the time, Savannah Haseler, insisted on ordering food for our table. Servers appeared bearing platters of contraband: breaded chicken wings with pimiento cheese grits, smoked pork trotter mac-and-cheese fritters, black-eyed pea chipotle hummus, Southern beer nachos, cornmeal-fried trout, and pitcher after pitcher of local craft beer. I sipped my soda water, picked at a small plateful of mixed salad greens, and snagged a few grilled shrimp as the serving platter came around.

I came away from Twain's without breaking any of Hartwig and Urban's diktats. I wouldn't say tiger blood pulsed through my veins, but I did feel the surge of smugness. Surviving the evening of superhuman temptations strengthened my resolve. The rest of my Whole30 experiment was a snap. As the days went by, my pants began to fit more comfortably. My shirts no longer strained at their buttons. On the thirty-first morning, I stepped on my bathroom scale for the first time in a month. Maybe I wasn't glowing, but I did look better, and I had lost twelve pounds.

And then I promptly regained every one of them.

From their book-cover photographs, Hartwig and Urban, who have since divorced, seemed pleasant enough: in their forties, both thin, fit, and strikingly attractive. Definitely glowing. But exactly who were these people forbidding me and millions of other Whole30-ers to have cream in our coffee, a slice of artisanal bread, or a bowl of chili? More important, what qualifications did they have to claim that a healthful diet could include a lot of fatty beef and as many as five eggs at a sitting (a normal Dallas Hartwig breakfast) but no whole grains—recommendations that fly directly in the face of what the US Department of Agriculture (USDA) says constitutes a healthful diet?

Although they say that their program is backed up by "science-y stuff," little in their educational and professional backgrounds qualifies Hartwig and Urban as experts in nutrition and health. Hartwig, who grew up in British Columbia, graduated with a master's degree in physiotherapy from Andrews University, a small college in Michigan. Urban received a business degree through a satellite campus of the University of New Hampshire. In an interview with the *Telegraph*, the paper of her hometown, Nashua, New Hampshire, she said that she "went off the rails in college," becoming addicted to "every powder, pill, and chemical substance I could get my hands on. I lied. I stole. I was fired from my job. . . . I was a terrible person." While in drug rehab, she quit smoking and became obsessed with exercise. She and Hartwig met at a fitness center that he managed in New Hampshire, and together they decided to eat a more healthful diet that eliminated potentially harmful foods. They eventually moved to Salt Lake City because of its size and proximity to mountain hiking and skiing trails. There, they opened a strength-training and conditioning gym that they closed in 2009 to focus on what would become the Whole30.

So, what scientific validity does the Whole30 have?

Very little, it turns out. Laura Kerns, a clinical dietitian and public health authority at University Medical Center New Orleans, told me that Whole30-ers lose weight for the same reason that everyone who sticks to any diet that calls for the elimination of entire food groups loses weight: they consume fewer calories. There is virtually no way, she says, that you can eat enough meat, fruit, and vegetables to make up for the calories you forgo when you drop grains, legumes, sugar, dairy, and booze. And as I discovered, the flip side is that as soon as you resume eating normally, those lost pounds come charging back.

But the reappearance of my love handles was the least worrying aspect of the Whole30. According to a survey of nutrition experts, conducted by *U.S. News & World Report*, who looked at thirty-five popular diets and rated them on effectiveness for weight loss, ease of following, compliance with accepted nutritional standards, ability to combat heart disease, and possible health risks, the Whole30 ranked near the bottom.

There had been no independent scientific studies on the Whole30, but Kerns said that eliminating grains and dairy for a month dramatically reduces intake of calcium and B vitamins such as thiamin, riboflavin, folate, and niacin—a particularly bad idea for me, given that Doctor Dennis has me take a daily capsule of niacin to control my blood pressure. Without legumes and whole grains, my fiber intake decreased, which may have explained that constipation. Some studies show that fiber also helps lower cholesterol and may help prevent heart disease, type 2 diabetes, and obesity. Fiber also helps increase "good" bacteria in the gut that fight inflammation. Fermented dairy products, such as yogurt, benefit intestinal bacteria, which fight infection and obesity. It is well known that limited amounts of red wine can also lessen the risks of developing cardiac disease.

Experts contend that the psychological underpinnings of the Whole30 may set up followers for long-term failure. A paper by Yaguang Zheng, of Boston College, in the *International Journal of Obesity* concluded that dieters who weighed themselves on a daily basis (forbidden by the Whole30) lost more weight than those who got on the scales less often. The Whole30's unforgiving strictness is also absolutely unnecessary. According to the CDC, 99 percent of all people trying to lose weight experience lapses. But the occasional slip is no problem at all and can actually be a valuable learning experience, provided you make amends later. Hartwig and Urban's drill-sergeant approach to eating and the short duration of a Whole30 diet can set up participants to fail or return to their bad old ways after they have completed a Whole30 tour of duty. I consider myself Exhibit A in support of that contention.

Like Atkins, South Beach, the Zone, and dozens of others before them, the Whole30 is one of a continuous stream of diet fads to have swept the country. According to Marketdata Enterprises, the weight management industry in the United States raked in more than $72 billion in 2019 (more than the value of all the produce sold here). Each year, more than 45 million Americans buy nearly $500 million worth of diet and fitness books. Amazon lists nearly 40,000 titles in those categories. Dieters spend up to 80 percent more on their food than those who stick to their normal eating habits.

As my month as a Whole30-er so clearly demonstrated, diets almost never work over the long term. In many ways, dieting is a multibillion-dollar scam. Yes, if dieters have the discipline to stick with their regimens (a big if), they do lose weight. Yet research shows that the vast majority of dieters gain all their pounds back, and sometimes more. In a 2007 *American Psychologist* article, Traci Mann, head of the Mann Lab at the University of Minnesota, conducted what still is one of the most comprehensive analysis of research on diets, looking at the results of thirty-one long-term studies—every study she could find that followed dieters for between two and five years. Mann showed that dieters typically lost between 5 and 10 percent of their body weight initially (as I had), but after two years, 83 percent had gained back more weight than they had lost. One four-year study of 19,000 older men (my bracket, once again) showed that one of the best predictors that participants would *gain* weight in the future was their having been on a diet at some point before the study started. The dieters were worse off than a control group, who ate whatever they wanted. Scientists have known about the futility of dieting for seven decades. In 1959, researchers conducted a review of all studies on weight loss conducted over the previous thirty years and came to one conclusion: diets simply did not work. Period. "We've spent decades counting calories, eating fat-free foods, sweating it out at the gym, and testing our willpower, and where has it gotten us?" wrote David Ludwig, of Harvard Medical School, in his 2016 book, *Always Hungry*. "We are a nation of dieters, and the diet isn't working. Most current strategies to battle obesity appear doomed to fail."

By any measure, I failed the Whole30—or maybe the diet failed me. Within a few weeks after my month of deprivation, I gradually went back to eating the same foods I had consumed before and weighed the same as I had on day one. But I was also left with that pledge I had made to myself in Doctor Dennis's office. How was I going to lose my forty unwanted pounds?

CHAPTER TWO

INSTANT RESULTS

I owe Doctor Dennis an apology. When I told him about my plans to search for a weight-loss program that worked, he asked me to promise not to try anything stupid. He said that slimming down was a worthy goal, so long as it did not pose obvious health risks. Despite everything I knew, my desire to burst out of the starting gate with instant results triumphed. After an initial success, I reasoned, I would find a responsible eating plan that I could live with for the long term.

Coincidently, I had packed on even more pounds than usual during the recent holiday season. What better opportunity would I have to do a cleanse, a regime that allegedly would wash away the toxins and extra pounds that had accumulated in my body after a couple of weeks of unfettered Yuletide indulgence? A cleanse, I read, would also miraculously strip away up to twenty pounds—half of my weight-loss goal—in just ten days.

I chose a program called The Master Cleanse, which was invented in the 1940s but is enjoying a revival among celebrities like Beyoncé Knowles, who went on it when she needed to rapidly drop weight for her role in the 2006 film *Dreamgirls*. Numerous online sites sell books and Master Cleanse kits. YouTube videos about cleansing abound. Dieters gulp down $200 million worth of bottled juice cleanses each year. One in five adult Americans who want to lose weight has tried a cleanse. I figured that any diet good enough for Beyoncé was good enough for me.

The regimen is simple. According to The Master Cleanse website, I could consume no food. My "diet" would consist of water and six to twelve glasses per day of a lemonade concoction made up of two ounces of lemon juice (hence its nickname, "The Lemonade Diet"), an equal amount of "robust" maple syrup, and a dash of cayenne pepper. Each morning and evening I was instructed to drink an herbal tea laxative called Smooth Move, which the site said would allow my bowel movements to remain "liquid and runny."

I would never have attempted a Master Cleanse had I taken a little time to run the most rudimentary background check on the quack who developed it. Stanley Burroughs was a handsome, wavy-haired Midwesterner who moved to Portland, Oregon, in the 1930s to trade in lumber. Declaring that he wanted to become famous, Burroughs abandoned that business to become an alternative medicine practitioner, first in California and later in Hawaii. In addition to prescribing his "lemonade"

THE MASTER CLEANSE

FOR UP TO 40 DAYS,

MORNING AND NIGHT

NO SOLID FOOD

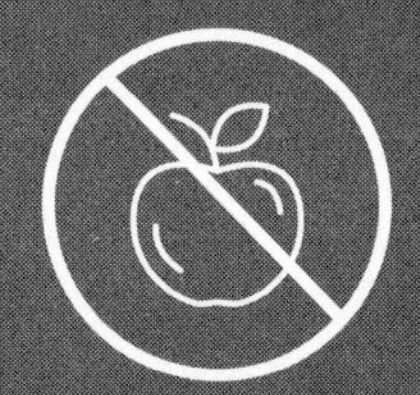

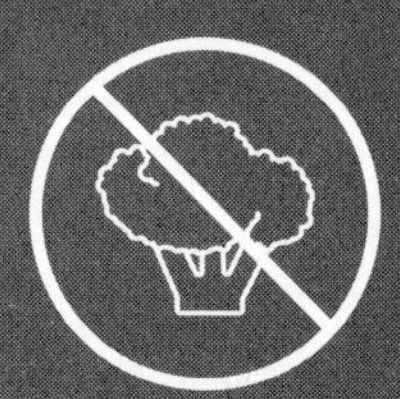

6–12 GLASSES OF LEMON JUICE AND MAPLE SYRUP, IN EQUAL PARTS, MIXED WITH WATER SEASONED WITH CAYENNE PEPPER.

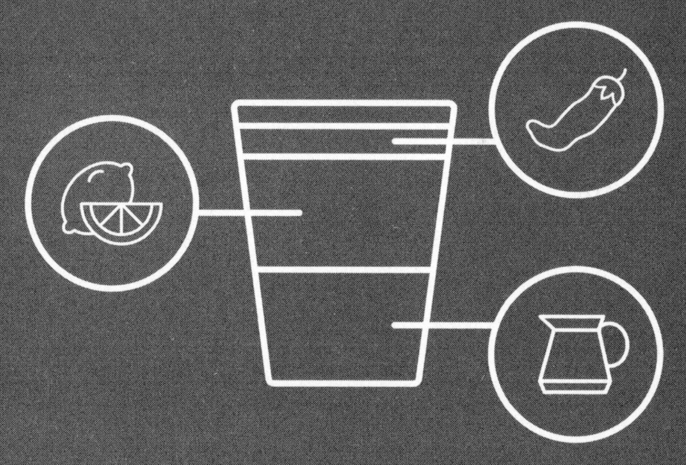

1 CUP LAXATIVE TEA

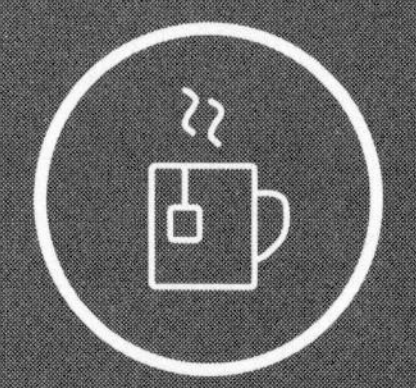

diet, he also treated patients by exposing them to light of various colors and through deep massage and reflexology, the practice of applying pressure to the feet, hands, and other parts of the body. Over the course of his career, he racked up felony convictions for practicing medicine without a license and failure to pay support to his ex-wife and three daughters. He barely escaped a prison sentence for manslaughter after one of his patients died of a massive abdominal hemorrhage following a massage session. Doctor Dennis would have been appalled.

In his book *The Master Cleanser*, which he began to distribute in the 1950s, Burroughs made it clear that his program was meant to be far more than a way to quickly shed a few unwanted pounds. "This diet will prove that no one needs to live with disease," he boasted. "Lifetime freedom from disease has become a reality."

He argued that illness, old age, and death were caused by poisons that accumulated in the body and were stored in "lumps and growths" that form in the lymphatic glands, liver, spleen, colon, stomach, and heart. The only way to eliminate these toxins, he claimed, was to go on his lemonade diet, which he contended could be "used with complete safety for every known type of disease." Participants could stay on it for as long as forty days. It would remove cholesterol from the bloodstream and dissolve plaque deposits in the arteries. Boils, abscesses, and all other skin disorders would disappear. It could cure stomach ulcers. Smokers, drug addicts, and alcoholics would lose their cravings. As a bonus, the lemonade diet was "superior in every way to any other weight-reducing diet." Lemons, according to Burroughs, were the richest source of minerals and vitamins of any food. Pure maple syrup was the most perfectly balanced sweetener. Cayenne built up blood supply and broke up mucus, thus hastening the elimination of toxins.

It was all bunk, as ridiculous as his claim to have the ability to levitate himself.

To give him some credit, he warned that there were downsides to cleansing. Participants might feel dizzy and agitated or weak. Vomiting and joint pain were not uncommon. But he insisted (wrongly) that these symptoms were caused by poisons leaving the body—sure signs that the diet was working its magic.

Since one of my hobbies is tapping maple trees in the forest behind our house each spring, I always have a ready supply of maple syrup. It seemed karma had predestined me to try The Master Cleanse. On my first morning, I combined two ounces of maple syrup with an equal amount of freshly squeezed lemon juice and a dash of cayenne pepper in an eight-ounce glass of warm water. If you had to develop a recipe that amplified the most disagreeable traits of those ingredients, I don't think you could do better. The lemon contributed sourness that was almost unbearable. In contrast, the maple syrup was cloyingly sweet. Besides being uncomfortably hot, the cayenne lent a gritty mouthfeel to the beverage. The best I can say about it is that the drink left a taste in my mouth so loathsome that it obliterated any traces of hunger. Temporarily.

Within an hour, my stomach growled ferociously. As instructed, I sated myself with another palate-numbing drink and repeated the process four more times that day. The only variety in my diet was a Smooth Move laxative tea, sipped just before bedtime.

I began day two with another Smooth Move and more hunger pangs. Although I downed my lemonade drinks, I could think of nothing but food and eating. My sense of smell went into overdrive, and it required all the steely resolve I could muster to walk past the door of a local lunch counter with its aromas of frying hamburgers, melted cheese, cake, muffins, and coffee, on my way to the post office and bank.

On day three, the cravings continued and were compounded by the effects of my Smooth Move teatimes. I guess that the manufacturer's marketing department believes that Smooth Moves is a more socially palatable brand name than Watery Moves, which would have been much more accurate. The resulting diarrhea was controllable at first, but after one desperate sprint to the toilet (barely avoiding the unthinkable), I had to station myself within a few strides of the bathroom. I don't want to imagine what would have happened if I had been driving my car, socializing with friends, or attending a business meeting.

By day four, being tethered to the toilet no longer mattered. I felt so faint and dizzy that I couldn't have moved very far even if I had dared to. I became frightened that I would fall, pass out, or worse. Per the website's recommendation that I return to solid food slowly, and with Doctor Dennis's warning that I not do anything stupid playing in my head, I opened a can of minestrone soup.

Yes, by limiting myself to less than 1,200 calories a day (about half of the USDA's recommended intake for a man my age and size), I had dropped seven pounds in less than a week. All of which promptly returned within days after I bade good-bye to maple-flavored lemonade and steaming cups of Smooth Move.

"Your body was sending you a message," said Liz Applegate, the distinguished senior lecturer emerita in the Department of Nutrition at the University of California, Davis, when I described the dizziness and lethargy I began feeling toward the end of my cleanse. "Three days is not a big deal, but after that, problems can develop, especially if you are older—in your forties, fifties, sixties—or if you are prediabetic, a condition you might not be aware of."

Applegate explained that during the cleanse, my body was doing everything it could to get glucose (a sugar that is an important energy source for the body) to my brain. But because of my very low calorie intake, the task became overwhelming, and my mind was not working as well as it could, resulting in that lethargy and dizziness.

The Master Cleanse provides virtually no protein, which is necessary to maintain a healthy immune system. "People, particularly older people, need a steady supply of protein. Lack of it can cause immunological effects and leave you vulnerable to bacteriological infections and upper respiratory infections," she said.

"When you stop eating, your body can undergo a massive shift in levels of electrolytes," she explained. Electrolytes are minerals such as sodium, calcium, and potassium. Think of them as the body's electrical wiring. They help transmit nerve impulses that allow muscles (including the heart) to contract and relax. They also maintain the balance of water inside and outside of cells as well as the balance between acids and bases in the blood. Improper electrolyte levels can cause abnormal muscle and kidney function and irregular heartbeat. In extreme cases, electrolyte imbalance can be fatal.

A recent study, Applegate said, showed that participants on a cleanse saw blood levels of HDL ("good cholesterol") decrease and experienced an increase in levels of homocysteine, an amino acid that can damage the insides of blood vessels, causing them to become narrower, which can result in heart attacks or strokes.

Applegate told me that my rapid weight loss was caused by two conditions: When you go without food, your body gets its energy from glycogen, which is stored in the liver and muscles. Glycogen is bound to water. When glycogen is burned by cells, the water once associated with it is released and gets flushed away in the urine. Many of my vanishing pounds were that water. Once I began to eat again, my liver and muscles went into overdrive to rebuild their glycogen supplies and the water associated with them. I owed much of the rest of my weight loss to the diarrhea brought on by those cups of laxative tea and the cayenne in the lemon–maple syrup concoction. Cayenne can irritate the colon (another reason people with sensitive bowels should not cleanse), and water is drawn there to wash away the irritant.

It turns out that cleanses do not cleanse at all. "Your body does a wonderful job of cleansing itself," Applegate said. The liver, kidneys, and intestines are highly capable of ridding our bodies of toxins on their own. "Mother Nature figured that out a long time ago."

CHAPTER THREE

DIET NATION

The Master Cleanse and Whole30 provided me with one lasting benefit: I was equipped with firsthand knowledge and a healthy mistrust of the culture of going on diets, particularly fad diets. Before venturing back into the weight-loss world, I vowed that I would make myself an educated consumer of dietary advice. As a journalist, I had spent my career imploring readers to learn how their food is produced before deciding whether or not to allow it on their tables—to be mindful eaters. I even spent a couple of years as the editor of *Eating Well* magazine, which is all about healthful food. I should have known better.

When it came to taking a step that could have had serious consequences for my health, I ignored my own advice by jumping on the Whole30 and Master Cleanse bandwagons with no more thought than I put into buying a bag of onions. It was a mistake I did not want to repeat.

I would refrain from going on another long-term diet until I had read academic research and interviewed nutritionists, doctors, and scientists who could explain what effect the foods I was or wasn't eating would have on my body. I wanted to know how and why the pounds were coming off—if indeed they were. What were the potentially harmful side effects? I wanted to make sense of all the contradictory scientific advice that seems to change monthly as reporters rush to interpret the most recent journal articles. Is fat evil? How about sugar? What about white flour?

But even the most scientifically sound diet is no good if it's too onerous to follow. Would I be hungry all the time? Would I experience lightheadedness? Irritability? Bowel issues? Could I accommodate the diet to my usual routines, which include frequent airplane flights, dinner parties, and visits to restaurants? To answer these questions, I planned to test-drive several common diets simply to see whether I could sustain the eating styles they championed, or whether they, like the Whole30, would be too extreme to adopt for the long haul. I have no scientific or medical background whatsoever, unlike many authors of diet books, and I consider a lack of bias and reporting experience to be my major qualifications to write this one. Nutrition experts cling dearly to their theories—understandable in that the most prominent of them have spent decades doing research, and their professional reputations are on the line. Me, I didn't care. I just needed to lose weight. I had no horse in the race other than my rotund belly. Besides, if I could find a way to lose weight after an adulthood defined by chubbiness and a spotty record in the willpower department, then anyone could.

The Master Cleanse is only one player in the grand old American tradition of diets that have been promoted by a series of unscrupulous quacks, kooks, and hucksters to a populace desperate to lose weight and willing to try anything that promises quick, painless results. In the late 1980s, the Health, Weight, and Stress Clinic at Johns Hopkins University compiled a list of nearly 29,000 weight-loss schemes that had been foisted on the country at one time or another. Most of them were junk (94 percent, according to the head researcher of the Johns Hopkins project) if not downright fraudulent.

As early as 1935, Carl Malmberg—who edited the magazine *Health and Hygiene* before becoming the chief investigator for the U.S. Senate Subcommittee on Health and Education—authored a book entitled *Diet to Die*. In his slim but prescient volume, Malmberg presented a reassuringly level-headed indictment of the dieting phenomenon. His words still ring true more than eight decades later. "No single subject, with the probable exception of religion, has grown up around it a larger body of error, misinformation, and plain buncombe than the subject of diet," he wrote. "Probably no field has been so thoroughly exploited by these self-styled scientists as that of food and diet. Nowadays, no doctor intent upon getting his name before the public by promulgating a new system of diet would fail to lay the greatest stress upon the scientific nature of his system, even though it might be so unscientific as to be immediately suspect to a layman with some knowledge of the subject." (Reading that reminded me of the Whole30's authors' claim that their program was based on "science-y stuff.")

Nonetheless, for the better part of two centuries, Americans have been suckers for all manner of wacky eating schemes. In retrospect, many now seem ludicrous, even humorous, but any modern dieter should consider them in perspective: At the time of their popularity, millions of desperate, overweight people slavishly followed them. Their creators were viewed as nutrition experts, and many became famous and wealthy. It's no different today. When you go on a diet, you and your health are entering this gonzo world. It's quite possible that in a few decades, the diet you go on today will be looked upon with the same ridicule we view the schemes of the past, an unfortunate number of which deserve our contempt.

In 1895, Horace Fletcher, a wealthy San Francisco businessman, was refused life insurance because of his weight. At forty years of age and standing only five feet seven inches tall, he weighed 205 pounds. To get back in the good graces of the insurance company, he lost 42 pounds. The key to his leaner body, according to Fletcher, was that he chewed every morsel of food until it became devoid of taste and completely liquefied. Fletcher insisted that if food retained a trace of flavor, it was not ready to be swallowed. He spat out any solids that did not succumb to the persistent grinding of his molars. Diners, he said, should chew at a steady rate of 100 times per minute. Each food item demanded a different number of carefully tallied chews. A bite of toast could be swallowed after 30; a single shallot required 722. Thorough mastication prevented "putrid decomposition" in the stomach and farther down the alimentary system. Fletcherites, as he called his followers, defecated less often and less offensively. The Great Masticator himself had but one bowel movement every two weeks, weighing between two and four ounces. In his own words, his "digestion-ash" was "no more offensive than moist clay" and no more odiferous than a "hot biscuit." He often carried samples around to silence doubters.

Fletcher had a discomforting obsession with defecation:

> Masticate all solid food until it is completely liquefied and excites in an irresistible manner the swallowing reflex or

> swallowing impulse. Attention to the act and appreciation of taste are necessary, meantime, to excite the flow of gastric juice into the stomach to meet the food.
>
> Strict attention to these two particulars will fulfil the requirements of Nature relative to the preparation of the food for digestion and assimilation; and this being faithfully done, the automatic processes of digestion and assimilation will proceed most profitably, and will result in discarding very little digestion-ash (fæces) to encumber the intestines, or to compel excessive draft upon the body energy for excretion.
>
> The assurance of healthy economy is observed in the small amount of excreta and its peculiar inoffensive character, showing escape from putrid bacterial decomposition such as brings indol and skatol [both compounds that make feces stink] offensively into evidence.
>
> When digestion and assimilation has been normally economic, the digestion-ash (fæces) may be formed into little balls ranging in size from a pea to a so-called Queen Olive, according to the food taken, and should be quite dry.

Promoted by the slogan, "Nature will castigate those who don't masticate," Fletcherism became an international craze. Society ladies held munching luncheons, where guests sat around tables wordlessly watching each other's jaws grind and timing their chewing with stopwatches. John D. Rockefeller, Franz Kafka, Henry James, and Thomas Edison became devoted Fletcherites. One Oklahoma senator proposed that all schoolchildren be taught Fletcherism. The Great Masticator claimed that if everyone followed his example, there would be no slums and no criminals. "In a single generation, the whole social problem would be solved," he said. Protracted chewing would also turn "a pitiable glutton into an intelligent epicurean." An additional benefit was that thorough chewing would deliver more nourishment to the body from a smaller amount of food, thereby saving followers money. And, of course, Fletcherites would lose weight. All that time spent chewing automatically decreased the amount of food swallowed and therefore calories consumed.

Fletcher had plenty of loony competitors in the early decades of fad dieting. A doctor from upstate New York, named James Henry Salisbury, became convinced while tending Civil War soldiers that the rampant diarrhea affecting the troops could be cured by a diet limited to ground beef. He later amended his beliefs to create the Salisbury System of Weight Reduction, which advocated a daily menu consisting of three pounds of rump steak, one pound of codfish, and three quarts of hot water. Salisbury completely forbade the consumption of vegetables and starches, convinced they produced toxins that caused coronary disease, tumors, and even insanity. Salisbury's name lived on, as I remember all too well. Once a week, my mother would feed us Salisbury steak, an overcooked, oblong, and slightly peppery hamburger patty drowning in gravy, which was a common entree in the frozen TV dinners that Mum served us in the family room. Dr. Salisbury would have been horrified to learn that the purity of his namesake main course was sullied by peas and mashed potatoes.

In his immodestly titled book *Eating to Banish Disease and to Save Civilization*, James Raymond Devereux took an approach to perfect health that directly contradicted Salisbury's. Writing in the early 1900s, Devereux prescribed a meatless diet of three meals a day—the first made up of only vegetables, the second only fruits, and the third only nuts. He stipulated that everything consumed should be raw. In unrelated (but equally perplexing) medical advice, Devereux also advised pregnant women to climb trees if they wanted easy deliveries.

The notion of separating food groups was taken to an extreme in a diet promoted by Dr. William Hay (whose Pennsylvania sanatorium was called the Pocono Hay-ven) and adopted by Henry Ford and other luminaries. In his 1929 book, *Health via Food*, Hay insisted that the way to remain slim was to never consume protein and carbohydrates during the same meal. He based his diet on the completely erroneous theory that carbohydrates were digested only in the mouth, and proteins only in the stomach. The body was incapable of performing both functions simultaneously.

In the 1920s and 1930s, the Hollywood diet, designed for actors and actresses who needed to slim down fast for film roles, became a national craze. Adherents consumed grapefruits and melba toast, supplemented with some lettuce, celery, tomato, and the occasional hard-boiled egg. On a typical day, those on the diet would eat the following:

BREAKFAST
— Half a grapefruit
— Melba toast
— Black coffee without sugar

LUNCH
— Half a grapefruit
— Melba toast
— Four celery stalks
— Black coffee without sugar

DINNER
— Half a grapefruit
— Half a head of lettuce
— One tomato
— Two hard-boiled eggs
— Black coffee without sugar

DIETING BY THE NUMBERS

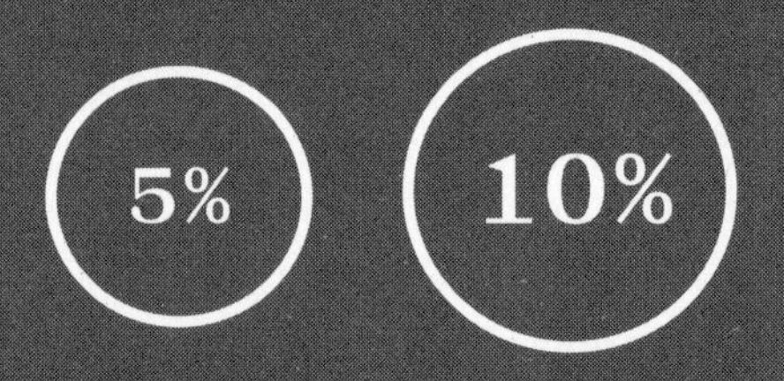

DIETERS LOSE BETWEEN 5 AND 10% OF THEIR BODY WEIGHT ON DIETS.

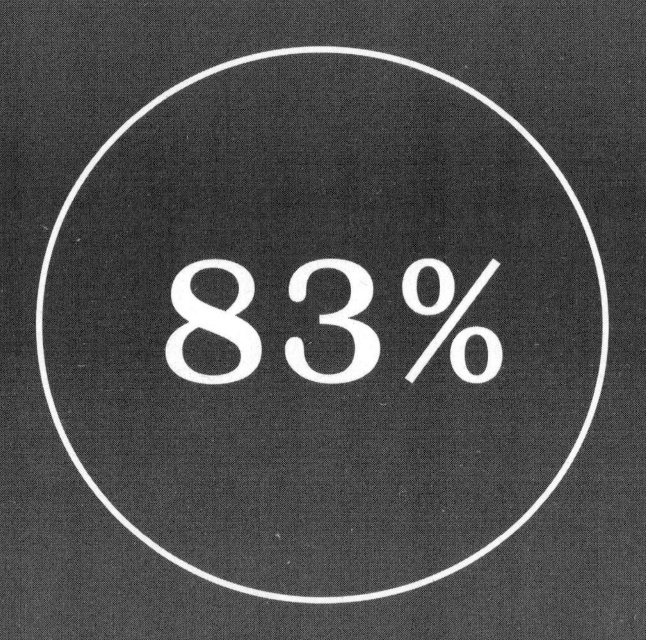

TWO YEARS LATER, 83% HAVE REGAINED THE WEIGHT PLUS ADDITIONAL POUNDS.

Despite its extreme limitations, this 600- to 700-calories-per-day diet became so popular that restaurants catered to its followers with special Hollywood dining options (at a higher cost than regular fare), and dinner-party hostesses fretted over what to offer guests on the diet, which should sound familiar to anyone who has tried to the navigate today's labyrinthine dietary restrictions when having guests over for a meal or trying to please returning adult children during the holidays. In *Diet to Die*, Malmberg wrote that there were "no figures on how many people literally killed themselves or became seriously ill by following the popular starvation diet, but it is certain that the toll was heavy."

In 1934, George A. Harrop, a respected physician associated with Johns Hopkins University, published a paper in the *Journal of the American Medical Association* touting the benefits of his banana and skim milk diet. The United Fruit Company (an ancestor of today's Chiquita brand) printed a pamphlet based on Harrop's theories and, with fulsome endorsement from the American Medical Association, distributed it nationally through doctors' offices. The diet restricted participants to four to six bananas and three to four glasses of skim milk a day, along with minimal amounts of roughage for a daily total of between 700 and 1,000 calories. Harrop's success spawned numerous two-ingredient imitators: diets allowing only tomatoes and hard-boiled eggs; pineapple and lamb chops; or baked potatoes and buttermilk.

And if two-ingredient diets worked, wouldn't a one-ingredient program strip off even more unwanted pounds? Even in the late 1800s, John Harvey Kellogg, the brother of the founder of the breakfast cereal company, put patients with high blood pressure on a diet of nothing but grapes—up to fourteen pounds of them a day (which would have added up to 4,200 calories). Actress Irene Rich vouched for a diet of grape juice in the 1930s (promoted by Welch's, of course). Ida Jean Kain, a popular writer and author of a syndicated newspaper column called "Your Figure, Madame!" contended in the 1940s that the key to losing two pounds per week was eating half a head of iceberg lettuce before each meal. After that, she said, the mere thought of eating an actual meal would become repulsive. Similar weight reduction results could be had by visiting one of the many "milk farms" across the country, where guests subsisted primarily on milk, augmented by orange juice and soup. In the 1920s, the cabbage soup diet swept the nation. You could lose twenty pounds a week and consume all the cabbage soup you wanted. There was one downside that limited the diet's popularity: participants reported that it produced unrestrainable quantities of weapons-grade flatulence. The next logical step was a no-ingredient diet. In the mid-1970s, newspaper stories reported that Elvis Presley kept his pelvis gyrating by going on the Sleeping Beauty diet, which recommended sedating yourself for days at a stretch, thereby losing the energy necessary to get out of bed and eat, let alone gyrate.

The diet industry even found ways for Americans to drop pounds while indulging in their favorite vices. During the 1920s and '30s, the American Tobacco Company, manufacturer of Lucky Strike cigarettes, ran an advertising campaign urging women to "Reach for a Lucky instead of a sweet." Ironically, the advice might have been effective, at least for weight loss. At that time, American Tobacco laced its cigarettes with appetite-suppressing chemicals.

My businessman father, along with many of the men in his social circle, eagerly embraced the advice of Robert Cameron, a San Francisco bon vivant whose fifty-page booklet, *The Drinking Man's Diet*, sold 2.4 million copies in the two years following its publication in 1964. "Did you ever hear of a diet that was fun to follow?" Cameron wrote. "A diet that would let you have two martinis before lunch and a thick steak generously spread with Sauce Béarnaise so that you could make your sale in a relaxed atmosphere and go back to the office without worrying about having gained an ounce? A diet that allows you to take out your favorite lady to a dinner of squab and broccoli with hollandaise sauce and Chateau Lafite followed by an evening of rapture and champagne?"

The secret was to drastically limit your intake of carbohydrates to sixty grams per day, about one-fourth the amount currently recommended by the U.S. Department of Health and Human Services' Dietary Guidelines for Americans. Booze, Cameron claimed (incorrectly), isn't particularly fattening when consumed while on his diet because high-protein foods stimulate an enzyme that metabolizes alcohol. He also put forth a wrong-headed theory that by dilating blood vessels, alcohol increased metabolism enough to compensate for the calories it contained. It's more probable that the drinking men lost weight because removing carbohydrates from the diet automatically deleted more than 1,000 calories a day for most of them. Critics today point out that the diet has too few carbohydrates to maintain good health, and all those well-marbled steaks are too high in saturated fat. As I recall, my dad did lose some weight. But a few years later he suffered a heart attack, a fate he shared with many of the men in his circle.

If all else failed, you could simply *Pray Your Weight Away,* as Charlie W. Shedd recommended in his 1957 book of that title. Shedd, a Presbyterian minister from Houston, dropped 100 pounds by praying to God, who, he believed, had designed humans to be slim. The obese, therefore, were by definition sinners who must turn to God for redemption. One of Shedd's imitators, Rev. H. Victor Kane composed a little prayer for divinely inspired dieters in his 1967 book, *Devotions for Dieters.*

I PROMISE NOT
TO SIT AND STUFF
BUT STOP WHEN
I HAVE HAD ENOUGH.
AMEN

Feel free to recite it and see if you lose weight.

CHAPTER FOUR

THERE ARE ONLY THREE DIETS

Most diets come and go. No one I know Fletcherizes. Nor have I met anyone who attributes his or her youthful figure to a milk-only diet, or a diet restricted to pineapples and lamb chops. But some early diets have become fixtures in our food culture. Their current promoters are clever enough to repackage them, tweak them a bit, and rebrand them with catchy new names to lend the appearance of novelty each time they come around again.

Nowhere is this more evident than in the constant recycling of two nineteenth-century diets that I have come to think of as the Jack Sprat and Ms. Sprat diets. The two types of programs both claim to produce weight loss and good health, but take diametrically opposed paths. Jack Sprat, as the nursery rhyme has it, "could eat no fat," and his followers say the correct way to diet is to eat carbohydrates and eschew meat, especially fatty meat. The adherents of his wife, who "could eat no lean," insist on the opposite: eat all the fat and meat you want, but avoid carbohydrates, especially the simple carbohydrates of sugars and processed wheat products such as bread and pasta.

The Jack and Ms. Sprat divide was made glaringly public in 2000 during a debate broadcast on CNN between two of the most famous diet titans of the late twentieth century. Dr. Dean Ornish, who lives on the West Coast, argued for a carbohydrate-rich diet with no meat and less than 10 percent fat. His opponent, Dr. Robert Atkins, whose offices were in Manhattan, advocated for eating few carbs and plenty of meat. But there was little new in either doctor's approach. Sixty-five years before the great diet debate, Carl Malmberg predicted in *Diet and Die*, "It is probably only a matter of time until we shall hear the battle between the starches and proteins dramatized and fought out."

A full century before Malmberg made his prediction, Jack Sprat first appeared on the nutritional landscape in the form of a Presbyterian minister named Sylvester Graham, who abandoned his pulpit and joined the Pennsylvania Temperance Society on a lecture tour to preach the gospel of bland food. With thick, dark hair and an exceptionally long nose, Graham fiercely warned that gluttony was the root of many social ills, including, but by no means limited to, violence and sexual intercourse. He completely banned meat. Insipid-tasting food discouraged excessive eating, in his view, and reduced the libido—a desirable effect. He also prohibited coffee, tea, salt, pepper, spices, sauces, and mustard. Instead, Grahamites were told to treat their stomach "like a well-governed child," and to eat vegetables, fruits, and nuts and drink only pure water.

He was particularly disdainful of yeast-leavened bread made with white flour, one of the foods, he believed, that led to rampant masturbation, especially among young people. God had ordained that wheat be consumed only in its whole, natural state, and that wheat products be made at home with a mother's hands, not in a commercial bakery. Additives used to whiten bread were sinful. Graham also distrusted yeast, which he accurately believed was a living organism. He, or one of his acolytes, devised a recipe for a whole-wheat, unleavened cracker that conformed to his standards and, with the help of s'mores and cheesecake crust, Graham's name lives on—the graham cracker.

The preacher's message began to gain national traction when the United States experienced a cholera epidemic that began in 1832. He blamed the outbreak, which first hit New York and other big eastern cities, on the urban sins of drinking alcohol and consuming meat and exotic foods. Graham noted that prostitutes and gay men who roamed the streets were particularly susceptible to the disease due to their sexual excesses and debauched lifestyles. (Cholera is actually caused by the bacteria *Vibrio cholerae* and transmitted through contaminated food and water.)

Graham became a celebrity, and his beliefs gained widespread acceptance. Followers launched *The Graham Journal of Health and Longevity*, which was filled with uplifting accounts of lives transformed by consuming bland food and no meat. Sufferers' indigestion, constipation, flatulence, and dyspepsia vanished overnight. As the fad spread, college students demanded that their cafeterias offer "Graham board." Hotel restaurants offering Graham-based fare opened in New York and Boston. Special stores sold only Graham-approved foods. Despite dutifully

GRAHAM-ISM

SYLVESTER GRAHAM

PRESBYTERIAN MINISTER IN THE 1800S

ALLOWED

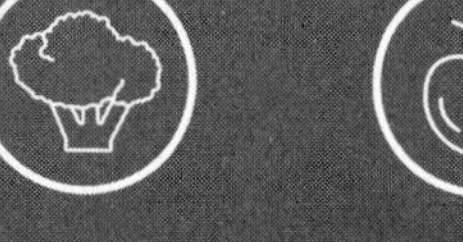

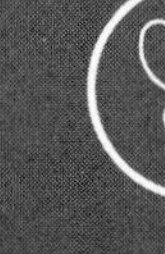
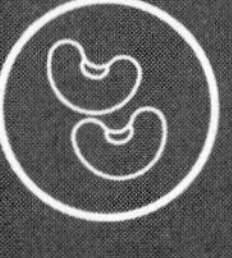

VEGETABLES

FRUIT

NUTS

WATER

NOT ALLOWED

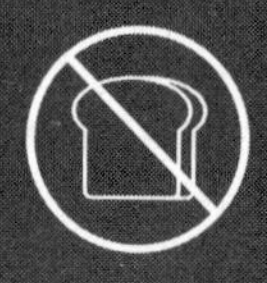

MEAT

COFFEE OR TEA

YEAST

SAUCES

MUSTARD

SPICES

SALT OR PEPPER

INFLUENCED

ORNISH DIET

PRITIKIN DIET

SEVENTH-DAY ADVENTIST DIETARY GUIDELINES

ESSELSTYN'S DIET

CHINA STUDY

practicing what he so fervently preached, Graham himself became sickly and died in 1851 at age fifty-seven.

But Graham-ism survived. In 1863, Ellen G. White, one of the founders of the Seventh-day Adventist church, collapsed on the ground during a service. When she regained consciousness, she proclaimed that, henceforth, church members would stop consuming meat, as well as alcohol, spices, sauces, tea, and coffee. Vegetables, fruits, and whole grains would replace them. Such a diet would lead to a healthy body and eliminate lustful urges such as masturbation, an abomination that she felt merited a death sentence. Sister White reported that God had given her these instructions while she lay in a trance on the floor, although it is obvious that either she or God borrowed heavily from the late Reverend Graham.

White and her husband, James, moved to Battle Creek, Michigan, in 1865 and founded the Western Health Reform Institute to apply their belief to patients who came there with digestive complaints. The institute gained a measure of professional stature in 1874, when a twenty-two-year-old doctor joined the team. His name was John Harvey Kellogg.

A Colonel Sanders–like figure who favored crisp white suits and white hats with brims—and was known to appear with a white cockatoo on his shoulder in public—Kellogg took to the institute's Graham-like principles with the zeal of a convert. During lectures, he asserted that coffee crippled the liver, tea led to insanity, and masturbation was the cause of cancers, poor vision, epilepsy, and diseases of the urinary tract. Kellogg was no hypocrite. He married a few years after taking up his post, but never had sex, even with his wife, Ella, who lived in the same house although they slept in a separate bedrooms.

Ella Kellogg did, however, recognize that patients soon grew weary of the monotonous meals served at the institute. To address that problem, she began tinkering with recipes that would conform to the diet's restrictions but impart a little flavor. One of her successes was to develop wheat-based flakes, which had the added benefit, in the Kellogg's opinion, of being an aphrodisiac. They became so popular among patients that the institute began selling them through mail-order and retail food stores. John Harvey Kellogg's younger brother, Will Keith Kellogg, or W. K., who was more business minded and less puritanical than his brother and sister-in-law, switched corn for wheat and added sugar to the flakes. The Kellogg Toasted Corn Flake Company evolved into today's Kellogg Company with $13 billion in annual sales and 34,000 employees. Its products are sold in 180 countries.

Graham-ism is alive and well. It lives on in Dean Ornish's books and in other recent bestselling diet programs that advocate low-fat, vegetarian fare, including Nathan Pritikin's *Pritikin Program for Diet and Exercise*, Dr. Caldwell B. Esselstyn's *Prevent and Reverse Heart Disease*, and T. Colin Campbell's *The China Study*—not to mention the twenty-one million members of the Seventh-day Adventist Church who are still encouraged to follow the dietary wisdom that the religion's founder received while she lay on the floor in a trance a century and a half ago.

William Banting, a retired English coffin maker whose deceased clientele had come from the upper echelons of London society, popularized the Ms. Sprat school of weight loss by eating mostly meat and fats. As Banting's business prospered, he steadily gained weight until in 1862, at age sixty-six, he carried 202 pounds on his five-foot-five frame. By then, his life had become unbearable: "I could not stoop to tie my shoe, so to speak, nor attend to the little offices humanity requires without considerable pain and difficulty, which only the corpulent can understand; I have been compelled to go down stairs slowly backwards, to save the jar of increased weight upon the ankle and knee joints, and been obliged to puff and blow with every slight exertion, particularly that of going up stairs."

For two decades, Banting had done everything possible to take off his extra pounds, which he compared to "the parasite of barnacles on a ship, if it did not destroy the structure, it obstructed its fair, comfortable progress in the path of life." He was hospitalized twenty times in as many years. One low-calorie diet caused him to break out in boils and carbuncles. On a doctor's recommendation, he began a daily rowing regime on the Thames. He became more muscular, but the exercise increased his appetite, and he put on weight even faster. "I have tried sea air and bathing in various localities, with much walking exercise; taken gallons of physic and liquor potasse [a potassium solution once thought to dissolve fat in obese individuals], advisedly and abundantly; riding on horseback . . . and have spared no trouble nor expense in consultations with the best authorities in the land, giving each and all a fair time to experiment, without permanent remedy, as the evil still gradually increased," he wrote.

When his sight and hearing began to fail, Banting consulted a doctor named William Harvey, who had recently been to Paris, where he learned about the theories expounded by Jean Anthelme Brillat-Savarin in his landmark book on the art of eating, *The Physiology of Taste or Meditations on Transcendental Gastronomy*. Although he may be better remembered today for quips such as "Tell me what you eat, and I will tell you what you are," Brillat-Savarin was an early proponent of a diet that eliminated starches, sugars, and anything made from flour.

Accordingly, Harvey advised Banting to give up bread, dairy products, sugar, beer, and potatoes because they contained "saccharine matter." But the doctor's orders were anything but Spartan. For breakfast, Banting could indulge in five ounces of beef, mutton, kidneys, boiled fish, bacon, or cold meat of any kind except pork. He could accompany his main courses with a cup of tea (no milk) and a piece of dry toast, which could be moistened with a little liquor. Lunch consisted of five or

WILLIAM BANTING

LONDON COFFIN MAKER AND SOCIALITE, INSTIGATED THE INTERNATIONAL TREND IN DIETING

NOT ALLOWED

BREAD

DAIRY

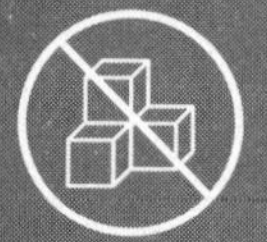

SUGAR

BEER

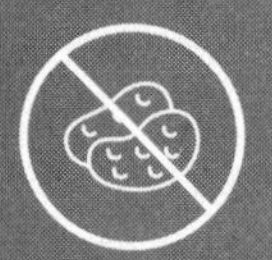

POTATOES

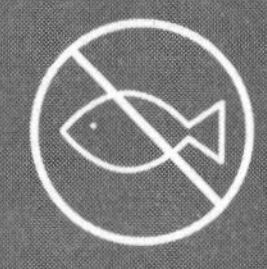

SALMON

SAMPLE DIET

BREAKFAST:
UNLIMITED MEAT, EXCEPT FOR COLD PORK, TEA, LIQUOR-MOISTENED TOAST

LUNCH:
POULTRY, FISH, VEGETABLES, 2–3 GLASSES FORTIFIED WINE

DINNER:
3–4 OUNCES MEAT OR FISH, 2 GLASSES WINE

BEDTIME:
1 GLASS WINE

INFLUENCED

ATKINS' DIET

SCARSDALE DIET

PALEO

THE ZONE

SOUTH BEACH DIET

WHOLE30

KETO

six ounces of any fish except salmon, any vegetable except potato, any kind of poultry or game, and two or three glasses of good claret, sherry, or Madeira. Dr. Harvey forbade port and beer. At teatime, Banting nibbled on a bit of fruit, ate a rusk or two, and had another cup of plain tea. Dinner consisted of three or four ounces of meat or fish and another glass or two of claret. Before retiring for the night, he was allowed to treat himself to either a tumbler of grog (gin, whiskey, or brandy) or another glass or two of claret or sherry, to bring his daily alcohol intake to between five and seven glasses of wine, on top of his liquor-moistened morning toast and that optional tumbler of grog.

The results, which Banting described as "simply miraculous," came almost immediately. He could stoop to tie his shoes. As the pounds disappeared, he was able to mount and descend stairs with ease. He once again easily performed all those "little offices humanity requires" and no longer suffered from indigestion and heartburn. He claimed that his eyesight and hearing improved. And, he lost forty-six pounds and twelve inches of girth over the course of a year. In Banting's case, the weight stayed off for the rest of his long life. "I have never felt better in health," he wrote.

To spread the good news, Banting published a booklet called *Letter on Corpulence Addressed to the Public*, which gave birth to the first international diet craze, as editions were published in Germany, France, Austria, Sweden, and the United States. He became known as "Mr. Banting of corpulence notoriety." For more than fifty years, his name was commonly used as a verb in the English language synonymous with dieting, as in, "I want to lose weight so I am banting." Banting himself lived for fifteen years after going on his famous diet, passing away at the venerable age of eighty-one. His legacy is the popular low-carb diet movement. Dozens of bestselling books expanded upon the concepts set forth in Banting's sixteen-page booklet. *Dr. Atkins' Diet Revolution,*

The Complete Scarsdale Medical Diet, The Zone, The South Beach Diet, The Paleo Diet, The Whole30, The Keto Diet, and many more owe their inspiration to the British coffin maker of corpulence notoriety.

The word *calorie* was nearly unheard of in the United States until 1887, when an American chemist named Wilbur Olin Atwater encountered the term while studying in Europe and brought the concept back home. By definition, a calorie has nothing to do with weight and dieting. It is simply a unit of measure. Just as pounds measure weight, inches distance, and gallons liquid, calories (which are called *kilocalories* by scientists) measure heat. One calorie is the amount of heat required to raise the temperature of one kilogram of water by one degree Celsius. Originally, the application of calories was limited to chemistry and physics, but by the mid-nineteenth century, European nutritionists began using calories to measure the energy values of different foods.

At first, Atwater concentrated on the number of calories required to fatten livestock, but he soon branched out to humans. In one experiment, he set out to discover the precise quantity of calories a bricklayer needed to eat each day to do his job. He attempted to popularize the term *calorie* in *The Century Magazine*, a mass-circulation publication based in New York, and through a series of papers published by the USDA. Photographs suggest that Atwater, a mustachioed man with puffy jowls and a bulging belly, apparently also enjoyed consuming more than the 2,830 calories per day that his own research showed was required for a man who took "light exercise."

Atwater viewed food as fuel—full stop. Something whose only value lay in giving a body, whether that of a cow or a human stone mason, the energy (or calories) required to grow, repair tissue, and move about as necessary. Consuming more calories than you needed, in Atwater's view, was borderline criminal. To provide adequate food to soldiers during World

War I, the government further publicized Atwater's research, admonishing Americans not to consume more calories than sustenance required. To exceed that would be detrimental to the war effort.

Eating too much would also run contrary to the cultural rage of the day. The end of the war coincided with a pivotal change in what Americans viewed as the ideal physique. Until then, a certain amount of rotundity on a man was a sign of vigor. For a woman, being buxom and hourglass shaped were considered attractive and evidence of robust health. But with the dawn of the flapper era, women aspired to develop lithesome, boyish figures. The new concept of counting calories was a foolproof, thoroughly scientific way to get rid of undesired pounds.

A California doctor named Lulu Hunt Peters introduced vast numbers of Americans to calories through the country's first blockbuster diet book. In 1918, Peters published *Diet and Health with Key to the Calories,* a slim manual intended both for those who wanted to *gain* weight as well as those who wanted to lose it. "The lack of knowledge of foods is the foundation for both overweight and underweight," she wrote.

Nonetheless, Peters's primary audience was clearly women who wanted to shed pounds. She had waged her own personal battles with obesity. "But cheer up. I will save you," she wrote in her mock-liturgical style. "Yea, even as I have saved myself and many, many others, so I will save you." She admitted that her ideal weight was 150 pounds, and coyly allowed that she was so thoroughly ashamed of her maximum weight that she would never reveal it, although she immediately told readers that there was once "seventy more pounds of me than there are now."

The book has more than its share of mathematical equations and complex tables listing the caloric value of foods. Peters also directed commands to her readers mercilessly. "Hereafter, you are going to eat calories of

CALORIE COUNTING

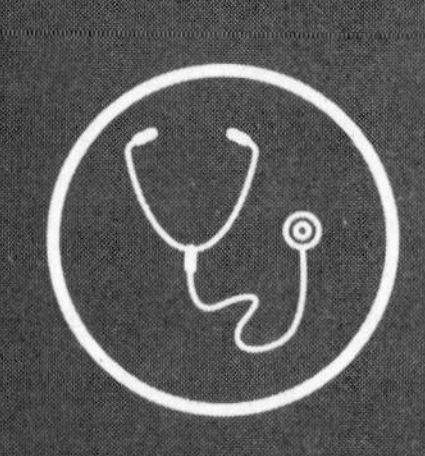

LULU HUNT PETERS

FEMALE PHYSICIAN AND AUTHOR OF AMERICA'S FIRST BESTSELLING DIET BOOK

INTRODUCED

HOW TO COUNT CALORIES

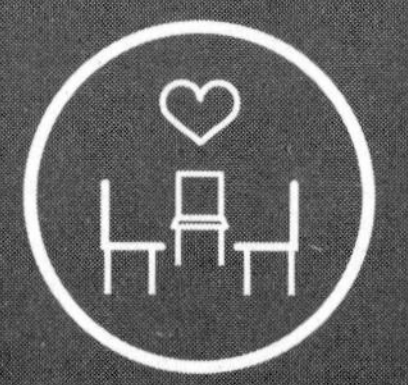

SUPPORT GROUPS FOR DIETERS

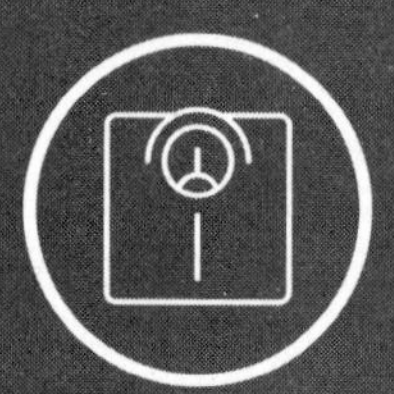

HOW CALORIES AFFECT WEIGHT LOSS AND WEIGHT GAIN

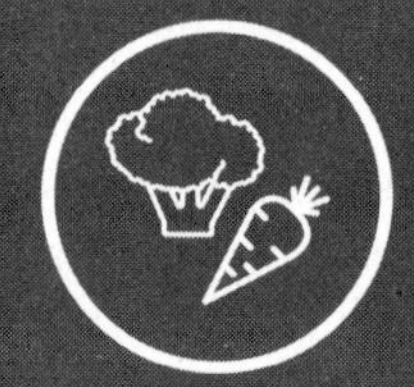

MANAGE HUNGER BY CONSUMING QUANTITIES OF LEAFY VEGETABLES

PRECURSOR TO

ATKINS' DIET

WEIGHT WATCHERS (WW INTERNATIONAL)

food. Instead of saying one slice of bread, or a piece of pie, you will say 100 calories of bread, 350 calories of pie," she wrote. She warned followers that they would always have to keep "watching their weight," thereby coining a term that would be taken up later by the Weight Watchers diet program, since renamed WW International. She drove home her message through hilarious, over-the-top prose—the sort of self-conscious narrative voice deployed by Laurence Sterne in his classic eighteenth-century comic novel, *Tristram Shandy*.

Early in *Diet and Health*, she insisted that any thin readers "Skip this chapter. It will not interest you in the least. I will come to you later. I am not particularly interested in you anyway. . . ." She issued similar instructions in the first paragraph of a later chapter called "At Last! How to Reduce," which she described as "strictly private and confidential, and is intended only for those who need it." In the next paragraph, she scolded any thin people who happened to be still reading.

Diet and Health, she said, was "illustrated by the author's small nephew Dawson Hunt Peters, the little rascal." She populated the book with imaginary characters with whom she had frequent verbal jousts. Their names were Mrs. Tiny Weyaton, Mrs. Knott Little, Mrs. Ima Gobbler, and Mrs. Sheesasite. In one passage, the unfortunately named Mrs. Weyaton asked, "We have heard you say that fat people eat too much, and still we eat so little?"

To which Peters replied, "Yes, you eat too much, *no matter how little it is*, even if it be only one bird-seed daily, *if you store it away as fat.* For hearken; food, and food only (sometimes plus alcohol) maketh fat. Not water—not air—verily, nothing but food maketh fat. (And between you and me, Mrs. Weyaton, just confidential like—don't tell it—we know that the small appetite story is a myth."

But she offered plenty of serious advice. Decades before Jean Nidetch came up with Weight Watchers, Peters urged readers to form groups to meet once a week and purchase a good set of scales for weigh-ins. She advised them to lose slowly and scientifically, and to keep from feeling famished by filling up on large quantities of leafy vegetables. She instructed them to read her food tables so they could "spend their daily calories wisely and carefully."

With millions of members in at least thirty countries, WW International is proof that the popularity of watching one's weight by tracking calorie intake remains popular. True, the company does not like to use the word *calorie*, replacing it with a simplified daily allotment of trademarked SmartPoints, which are based on the number of calories in food items, as well as saturated fat, sugar, and protein. But participants still monitor what they eat to stay below daily limits tailored to their weight. Other pay-to-lose commercial programs, such as Jenny Craig and Nutrisystem, ship customers prepared meals that are calorie restricted. And the fasting diets, such as the 5:2, in which participants eat normally for five days a week and severely limit food intake during the remaining two; or the time-restricted diets, where you eat everything within a restricted window of time each day, are also based on cutting—if not counting—calories.

So, who is right? Jack Sprat by not eating fat, Ms. Sprat by avoiding lean, or those who eat both fat and lean but monitor their caloric intake? The scientific literature is filled with papers supporting one approach over the others. And the creators of diets still argue vociferously for their plans. But one long-term study of more than eight hundred men and women on varying diet plans suggests that it all comes down to controlling calories. Dr. Frank Sacks, professor of cardiovascular disease prevention at Harvard School of Public Health, and his team divided the study subjects into four groups: those with a low-fat, average-protein diet; a

LOW-FAT, MEATLESS,
UNRESTRICTED CARBOHYDRATES

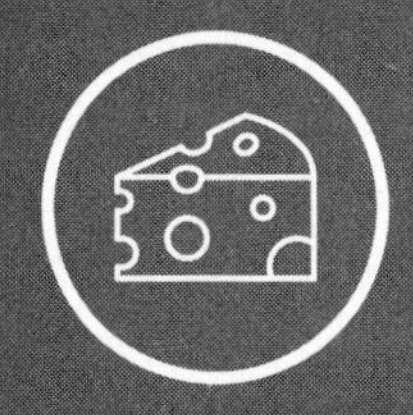
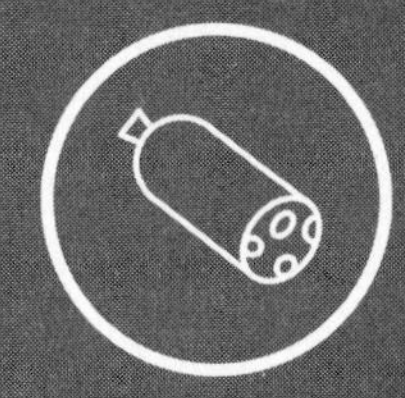
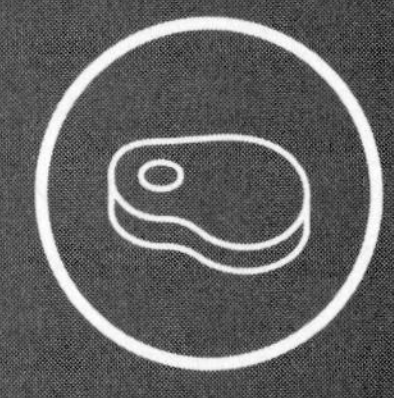

UNLIMITED MEAT AND ANIMAL FAT,
FEW CARBOHYDRATES

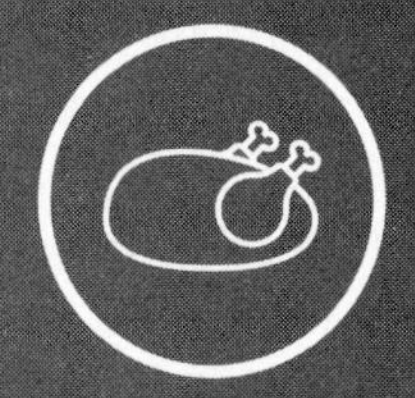

LIMITED CALORIC INTAKE

low-fat, high-protein diet; a high-fat, average-protein diet; and a high-fat, high-protein diet. Each participant was put on a diet that reduced calorie intake by the same amount—750 calories per day. The result, published in the *New England Journal of Medicine* in 2009, was that after two years, "weight loss and reduction in waist circumference were similar" for all four groups, implying that if you cut calories, you will lose weight regardless of the percentage of fat and protein in your diet. "These results show that, as long as people follow a heart-healthy, reduced-calorie diet, there is more than one nutritional approach to achieving and maintaining a healthy weight," said Dr. Elizabeth Nabel, director of the National Heart, Lung, and Blood Institute in a press release.

As the next step in my quest to lose weight, I decided to give three modern versions of the basic diets a try and interview their developers and other scientists, nutritionists, and medical doctors to see what was really happening to me. Was I destined to follow the path to slimness blazed by Graham (low-fat, meatless, plenty of carbs), Banting (lots of meat and fat, few carbs), or Peters (limit my calorie intake)—or none of them?

CHAPTER FIVE

DEAN CUISINE

A few years ago, two dozen of the world's leading nutrition scientists assembled for a summit in Boston. The gathering's ambitious purpose was to give the researchers the opportunity to sift through conflicting advice together and arrive at a consensus on what should constitute a healthful diet.

As one of a handful of journalists in attendance, I found it difficult to see how such a diverse group could agree on anything. Dr. S. Boyd Eaton, a patrician medical professor emeritus from Emory University, in Georgia, and considered the father of the popular paleo diet, expounded upon the virtues of eating an enormous amount of protein, vegetables, and fruit, while avoiding sugar, grains, and simple carbohydrates. For optimum health, we should, he said, mimic the diet of our preagricultural ancestors. Antonia Trichopoulou, regarded as the mother of the Mediterranean diet, had flown in from Athens, Greece, and advocated for her region's traditional cuisine, low in animal fat and high in olive oil and vegetables. Joan Sabaté, from Loma Linda University in California, claimed that vegetarian diets were far better than omnivorous diets for both the health of humans and the planet. David J. A. Jenkins, the Englishman who invented the glycemic index to rate foods on how rapidly the body converts the carbohydrates they contain into sugars, blamed simple carbohydrates for the current epidemic of heart disease and diabetes. Alessio Fasano, of Massachusetts General Hospital, in Boston, enlightened attendees about the perils of gluten. Harvard's Frank Hu, one of the members of the medical committee responsible for writing the 2015 Dietary Guidelines for Americans (the same guidelines that gave us the food pyramid of the 1990s), reported on a study showing that there was no association between the consumption of saturated fat and heart disease. His colleague Meir Stampfer disagreed, saying that eating red meat led to diabetes, cancer, and cardiovascular problems. Dr. Steven Abrams, chair of pediatrics at the Dell Medical School, at the University of Texas, in Austin, insisted that healthy diets for children, adolescents, and even adults should include milk and other dairy products. It was, one frustrated attendee observed, like witnessing the bickering among the learned elders in the parable "The Blind Men and the Elephant."

After a solid day of presentations and panels, the scientists reconvened in private over dinner to see if they could agree on the basic principles of healthful eating and communicate those findings to an understandably confused public.

To my surprise, when the bleary-eyed experts gathered in a conference room the next morning, they had, indeed, reached consensus. "The foods that define a healthy diet include abundant fruits, vegetables, nuts, whole grains, legumes, and minimal amounts of refined starch, sugar, and red meat, especially keeping processed red meat intake low," reported Dr. Walter Willett, of the Harvard School of Public Health, and the conference's co-chair. According to Willett, the scientists agreed to support the recommendations of the most recent version of the Dietary Guidelines for Americans, which emphasized fruits and vegetables, but placed no fixed upper limit on the amount of meat and fat in an optimum diet.

So, there it was. The first-ever broad agreement among world-famous nutrition scientists. Smiles broke out. The attendees nodded in unison. A self-congratulatory murmur spread through the room.

Then a hand shot up from the back row. A fit-looking man wearing a stylish black sport coat over a dark dress shirt and trousers stood. "I disagree," he said, his voice earnest, slightly high-pitched, and fast-paced, as if he was worried that he'd run out of breath before he made his point. "I want to go on the record as saying that what the dietary guidelines say about fat is not true." The room fell into an uncomfortable silence.

Dr. Dean Ornish has often found himself a lone dissenting voice against perceived wisdom in the medical community. In discussions about diet, Ornish has positioned himself on the extreme antifat fringe, promoting a diet based on fruits, vegetables, whole grains, legumes, and foods derived from soybeans. It contains less than 10 percent fat, including plant-derived fats, and no meat or animal products except egg whites, which are free of fat and cholesterol, and nonfat dairy products. He claims it is the "world's healthiest diet for most adults" and that adhering to such a diet can reverse heart disease. Low-fat advocates deify Ornish, but others who see simple carbohydrates, not meat and fat, as unhealthy, blame Ornish for contributing to the modern epidemic of diabetes, obesity, and heart disease. I thought it was worth hearing Ornish out, so I hopped a plane and flew across the continent to Sausalito, California, where he is based.

As a student at the Baylor College of Medicine in the mid-1970s, Ornish assisted in the operating room where renowned cardiac surgeon Dr. Michael DeBakey performed bypass surgery on the clogged arteries of patients' hearts. Although impressed with DeBakey's legendary scalpel skills, Ornish was disappointed by the ultimate outcomes of the delicate and costly procedures. Patients recovered from their operations, and immediately reverted to their former sedentary lives, smoking habits, and high-fat diets, only to return to the hospital a short time later once again in need of DeBakey's surgical talents. "Bypass surgery was the right term," Ornish told me when I met with him in his office. "The surgery *bypassed* the root causes of the problem. I thought, 'What if we went after the underlying causes of heart disease?' "

He found numerous studies that linked diets high in fat and cholesterol to high blood pressure and elevated levels of blood cholesterol, both risk factors for heart disease. Other research showed that stress could have the same effect. Conversely, exercise lowered the risk factors. But there were two huge holes in the science: No one had analyzed the combined effects of a low-fat, low-cholesterol diet; moderate exercise; and a program to reduce stress. Nor had anyone looked at how diet directly affected the buildup of arterial plaque, which is composed of fat, cholesterol, calcium, and other materials. Over time, it hardens and narrows arteries, which leads to heart disease.

Ornish brazenly decided that he was the one to fill in the gaps, even though he was still a few years short of getting his MD. Conducting the research and reporting his results would require dropping out of medical school for a year, much to the concern of his professors and hard-driving parents. As an experiment, he proposed to sequester a group of heart patients and, for one month, feed them a vegetable-based diet containing a maximum of 10 percent fat, less than one-third of the government's recommended level. In addition, his patients would exercise and practice yoga and meditation to reduce stress. He would go beyond the usual practice of measuring cholesterol and blood pressure. Instead he intended to measure the blood-pumping capacity of participants' hearts and levels of arterial plaque both before and after the study.

The medical world was unprepared for his revolutionary notions. This was an unenlightened time, when hospitals still had cigarette machines in their hallways, despite evidence showing tobacco's links to heart disease and cancer, to say nothing of the deep-fried, fatty offerings from their cafeterias. Ornish's professors thought he had lost his mind. There was no sense measuring arterial plaque, because everyone knew that coronary disease was cumulative and chronic. Once clogged with plaque, arteries only grew more clogged. There was no turning back the clock. As far as Ornish's hippie-ish yoga and meditation mumbo jumbo went, experts knew that, from the perspective of Western medicine, there was no such thing as a mind-body connection.

When Ornish told DeBakey about his proposal, the great man harrumphed and said, "What class are you in?" Learning that Ornish was a second-year student, DeBakey shook his head and said that was a pity. It would be hard to get a second-year candidate—even an obvious crackpot—kicked out of medical school. Other professors simply dismissed Ornish's ideas as utter nonsense. One doctor snidely asked if he was obligated to tell possible study subjects that he was referring them to a swami. Ornish's peers were equally scornful. "Do you really think that your mind can affect your body? What a stupid idea!" said one male classmate.

To which Ornish replied, "Have you ever had an erection?"

Despite the negative reactions that greeted Ornish's proposed experiment, Baylor had an enlightened policy of encouraging its students to undertake independent research, believing that they would learn valuable lessons, even from total failure, maybe especially from failure. Ornish scrounged up $5,000 in grant money, convinced Baylor to fund the necessary before and after heart scans, and, after being turned down by nearly every hotel in Houston, convinced the management at the Plaza to donate the use of ten rooms. He then assembled ten subjects, all of whom had chest pains, shortness of breath, and other serious symptoms of advanced coronary disease. They were so sick that Ornish had reason to fear that some might not survive the twenty-four-day regimen—a time span established because twenty-four days was the limit of the hotelier's generosity.

But it didn't even take the entire twenty-four days for participants on Ornish's low-fat, stress-reducing program to begin showing improvements. Patients formerly unable to walk across the street, go to work, or have sex without debilitating angina (chest pain caused by inadequate blood flow to the heart) reported a 90 percent reduction in discomfort. Scans showed that their arteries became less clogged. Their blood flow increased by 300 percent.

Ornish oversaw a subsequent five-year study that included a control group who consumed a diet that conformed to the government's 30 percent guidelines for fat intake. The subjects with low-fat diets showed an 8 percent reduction in artery blockages, while the others saw a 28 percent increase. The low-fat dieters also experienced a 91 percent reduction in strokes, heart attacks, bypasses, and angioplasties. Some literally got up out of their wheelchairs and abandoned their canes. Others successfully weaned themselves from prescription drugs to treat diabetes.

Today, Ornish, who is in his late sixties, is president of the Preventive Medicine Research Institute, a nonprofit scientific body he founded. He is also a professor of medicine at the University of California, San Francisco. He has been on the cover of *Newsweek* magazine, and *Life* magazine named him one of the fifty most influential members of his generation. He has authored more than seventy academic articles, which have appeared in such respected publications as the *Journal of the American Medical Association*, *Lancet*, and *American Journal of Cardiology*. All six of his books for general readers became bestsellers. Adherents to his diet and lifestyle recommendations range from entertainers such as Clancy Jones and Clint Eastwood to Silicon Valley highfliers, like the late Steve Jobs, to politicians such as Hillary and Bill Clinton. Even the previously hostile DeBakey telephoned Ornish and said, "I just wanted to thank you for keeping me alive all these years." The call came a few months before DeBakey's one hundredth birthday.

Ornish conducts his research and oversees programs in more than fifty hospitals and clinics nationwide, but the nerve center of his low-fat empire is a spacious office on the third floor of a building beside the harbor in tony downtown Sausalito. Except *downtown* does not accurately describe the quiet tree-lined streets and attractive low-rise architecture of the wealthy enclave.

The ceiling of Ornish's office was high and sloping, with exposed, barewood rafters. Spicy aromas drifted out of a test kitchen somewhere downstairs, where cooks developed recipes for his website. A friendly

DEAN ORNISH

PHYSICIAN, RESEARCHER, PROFESSOR OF MEDICINE

DO THIS

FRUITS

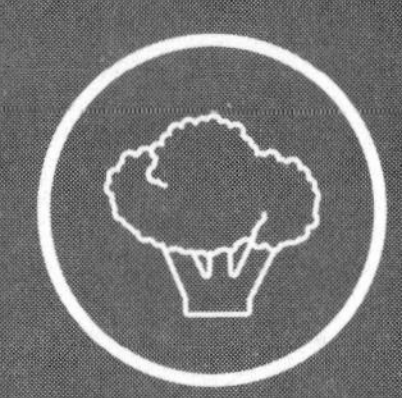

VEGETABLES

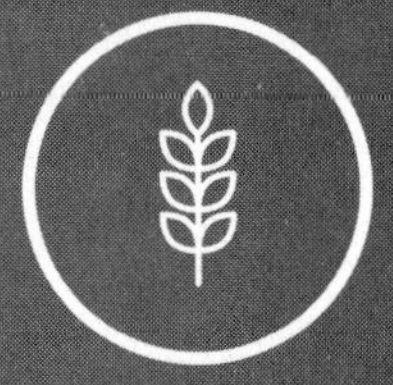

WHOLE GRAINS

SOY

CONSUME LESS THAN 10% FAT

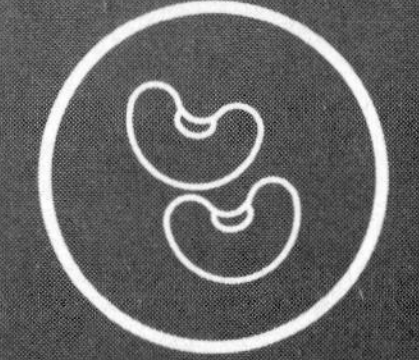

LEGUMES

NOT THIS

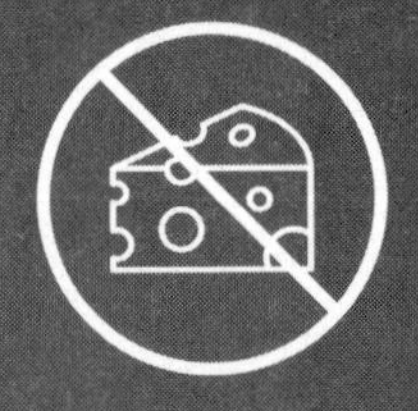

NO MEAT OR ANIMAL PRODUCTS, EXCEPT EGG WHITES AND NONFAT DAIRY PRODUCTS

French bulldog belonging to one of them apparently had the run of the place. Picture windows overlooked finger wharves, where sailboats and yachts were moored. Even though it was midmorning on a sunny, pleasantly warm day, few people were out, aside from the occasional jogger, dog walker, or cyclist. Normally raucous seagulls seemed mellow and respectfully low-key as they roosted on pilings or flapped lazily over the calm bay, with its fringe of luxury residences and mountain peaks. One of Ornish's walls was taken up by shelves filled with books and journals, often two deep. There were the usual work-space photographs of his wife and two kids. But the lasting impression of the space was that it served as a shrine for Ornish's many achievements: plaques, framed certificates, trophies, and photographs of Ornish and assorted celebrities and politicians, up to and including Barack and Michelle Obama.

He sat behind a curved, blonde-wood desk the size of a billiard table. Its surface was cluttered with a couple of laptops, two cell phones, a tablet, computer, and landline telephone, all of which he used while I was there, often simultaneously. Meeting with Ornish reminded me of having a "conversation" with my daughters when they were in high school and perpetually juggling a half-dozen discussions concurrently, far removed from me in space and time. He was perpetually on his cell phone, talking or checking email, and calling across the hall to his assistant's office.

He had flown home late the previous evening from Nashville, where he had been given the Lifetime Achievement Award from the American College of Lifestyle Medicine. It was the first time the award had been granted, he informed me. He woke up that morning at six o'clock and meditated for an hour before snuggling for a half-hour with his wife (number three) and daughter.

"She's such a sweet, happy girl. Our little love child," he said, smiling at the girl's photograph on his desk.

Ornish maintains a punishing routine. He breakfasted that morning on a bowl of whole-grain cereal and blueberries in low-sugar soy milk before dropping off his son at school and arriving at his office at about eight-thirty. When I got there at ten o'clock, he had just finished one conference call that had run over and was about to be connected to another. After that, he needed to talk to a doctor who wanted to bring the Ornish program to a hospital in Austin, Texas. Then he would rush across the bay to teach a class at University of California, San Francisco, before joining a meeting with fellow members of the American College of Cardiology's nutrition committee. That evening, he planned to attend a political fundraiser at the Napa Valley winery owned by Kathryn Hall, a former U.S. ambassador to Austria.

"This is after forty years of meditation," he told me, when I observed that his schedule sounded like the sort of crazy type-A pace that might be expected to cause heart attacks in men his age. "Today is not such a bad day," he said. "You should have seen me before. I couldn't sit down. I'm better than I was. Besides, type-A behavior is not harmful. It's when you accompany it with hostility and cynicism and anger. But I love what I do, and when I'm on my deathbed—hopefully at 150 years old—I want to look over my life and say that I made a difference. To create a whole new paradigm of preventive health care at a time when the medical system is so broken is really rewarding."

Ornish was born in Dallas. His father was a dentist, and his mother a historian and children's book author. As a boy, Ornish earned money as a magician, entertaining at birthday parties. By high school, his interests shifted to photography. Always precocious, he opened a professional studio and took wedding pictures. Later, he photographed rock stars for *Rolling Stone* magazine and wrote articles for *Esquire*, plum assignments most journalists could only wish for, even after decades of practicing the trade.

But for him, photojournalism was just a way to earn a bit of extra money. By the time he entered Rice University in 1972, he had decided to dedicate himself to a medical career, much to the relief of his parents, who, he said, had always sent him mixed messages about their professional expectations for him. "It was, 'We want you to do whatever makes you happy, but how could you do something that is different from what we want,' " he said. "Because they really didn't see me as being a separate person. That was a problem. That narcissistic thing where parents see their children as an extension of themselves."

But the chances of him becoming a doctor dimmed when Ornish attempted to clear the dreaded hurdle in every would-be doctor's path: organic chemistry. The professor who taught the course was a "cross between Adolph Hitler and the John Houseman character in the movie *The Paper Chase*," said Ornish.

"This is a weed-out course," the professor informed students on the first day of class. "And I am going to weed you out. You will never get to be a doctor unless you do well in this course." He required his students to memorize a vast quantity of chemical equations. Unfortunately, Ornish thinks analytically and conceptually rather than relying on the rote memory required by the class. He worried that he would fail, and as he tells it, that fear created a vicious cycle. In response, he became so agitated he couldn't sleep for days on end. He began drinking alcohol and taking tranquilizers. His memory losses became so severe he was unable to remember a newspaper headline five minutes after reading it, let alone convoluted formulas. It didn't help that his roommate had a photographic memory and got perfect grades without ever having to study. "The combination of feeling that I was never going to amount to anything because I was stupid, and that if I did it wouldn't matter because nothing could bring me lasting happiness was profoundly depressing," he said. "Everything lost meaning."

Ornish decided to commit suicide. At first, he planned to throw himself off an oil derrick near his Houston apartment, but realized his parents would be distraught knowing he had taken his own life. A more palatable option was to get drunk and fake an accident by intentionally slamming his car into a bridge abutment, a fate that would surprise no one who had ever driven with the teenage Ornish. The only thing that prevented him from carrying out his scheme was that a debilitating case of mononucleosis left him unable to get out of bed. His parents drove to Houston and brought him home to recuperate. Ornish had other ideas. "My plan was to go home and get strong enough to kill myself."

Help came in the form of a saffron-robed, white-bearded religious man called Swami Satchidananda, who had come to national attention as the man who sat cross-legged on the stage to open the Woodstock Music Festival. The swami's teachings had helped Ornish's sister overcome horrific migraine headaches; so in a gesture of gratitude, Ornish's parents invited Satchidanada to attend a cocktail party in their living room when he visited Dallas.

"There's an old saying that when the student is ready, the teacher appears, and that was certainly true for me," said Ornish. "Besides, I figured that I could always kill myself. I'll make that plan B. Let me try this weird stuff. And I began getting little glimpses of what it meant to be peaceful."

Ornish, who had always enjoyed a traditional Texan boy's diet, heavy on "cheeseburgers, steak, and deep-fried burritos," followed the advice of a meditation instructor and became vegetarian. He has not swallowed a morsel of meat since (he occasionally eats fish at a highly regarded sushi restaurant down the street from his office). He started to practice meditation and did stretching and breathing exercises, and soon became well enough to return to college. He graduated summa cum laude with a confirmed belief in the dietary and spiritual underpinnings of his future career.

During our discussion, Ornish frequently lapsed into soft-toned utterances that could have come out of the mouth of a swami. He said that real spiritual teachers are the ones who teach us to lead "joyful, pleasurable, meaningful lives, not lives of self-sacrifice." If you get your peace, health, and happiness from the outside world, then everyone and everything that has what you need has power over you. Pain and illness can be doorways to transformation. Great wisdom comes from making mistakes. At one point, he played a computer video of his daughter wearing colorful, oversized boots and spontaneously erupting into what he called a "happy dance" on a visit to Disneyland. "That dance captures the essence of what we want our wellness program to be," he said.

In stark contrast, Ornish's conversations about his work were often marked by a pronounced defensive tone, as if he were still trying to prove something to his demanding parents. He outlined his career through a series of well-rehearsed David-and-Goliath tales, casting himself as an underdog who, despite all odds, conquers the naysayers. Hidebound professors lined up against him, only to ultimately see the light. Ultratraditional Harvard academics viewed him as too young and inexperienced to conduct research under their institution's imprimatur, but the world's most respected medical journals published the results of research he did on his own. Administrators at the California Pacific Medical Center wouldn't agree with Ornish on how to divide grant money, forcing him to start the successful Preventive Medicine Research Institute, which he now heads. Bureaucrats in Washington dragged their feet for sixteen years before allowing Ornish's program to be covered by Medicare, succumbing only after a barrage of letters from the likes of Bill Clinton, Newt Gingrich, and Diane Feinstein (Ornish showed me a folder bulging with their correspondence).

He can become borderline vitriolic if the validity of his work is challenged. When I observed that even nutritionists who agree with his discoveries say that his program is too rigid for normal dieters to follow for any length of time, he all but barked that he had surveys showing that 85 percent of those who enter his program stick with it, a far higher rate than those who faithfully take prescribed heart medications. Detractors ignore that research, he said. To drive that point home, he turned on his laptop to show a video of a retired San Francisco restaurant owner named Mel Lefer who, after a life of cigars and rich food, suffered a major heart attack that left him unable to walk for more than two or three paces. Lefer was accepted in a year-long clinical trial run by Ornish, even though doctors doubted he would live for a year. Strolling briskly across his hilly back-yard in the video, Lefer tells the camera, "That was twenty-five years ago."

"I've got thousands of cases like this," Ornish said.

Yet in the last couple of decades, there has been a backlash against the fat-is-evil dogma he extols. One of Ornish's most formidable popular critics is journalist Gary Taubes, who ushered in the anti-Ornish movement in a famous 2002 cover story in the *New York Times Magazine* entitled "What If It's All Been a Big Fat Lie?" The cover photo was a fat-oozing, well-charred T-bone topped with a melting pat of butter. Taubes subsequently detailed his message that high-fat diets are fine in the 2007 book *Good Calories, Bad Calories* and, unusual for a nonscientist, has published articles in highly respected publications, such as *BMJ* (formerly the *British Medical Journal*).

Taubes makes a compelling case that carbohydrates, not fats, are the cause of obesity, diabetes, and heart disease. He contends that starchy potatoes, white flour, refined rice, pasta, and sugar make you fat, the accepted nutritional wisdom until the middle of the twentieth century.

He notes that there is a direct link between the 1980s, years when we dutifully began following the advice of medical experts and lowering our fat intake, and a spike in heart disease and obesity. Taubes points out that between 1960 and 1980 about 13 percent of the American population was obese, a figure that remained stable. But since then, even as we consumed less red meat and fat as a percentage of our caloric intake (and more carbohydrates), the obesity rate has surged to more than 30 percent. Taubes went so far as to suggest that ultra-low fat diets such as Ornish's actually drove up the levels of small, dense particles of LDL cholesterol (the "bad" kind) in our blood and could create a greater risk of heart disease.

"Taubes," Ornish, told me dismissively, "is a nonphysician. His books and articles contain no science other than what he chooses to report. My research shows that a low-fat diet can reduce the actual plaque buildup on artery walls. It's this buildup that can lead to heart attacks."

A low point for Ornish came in the middle of 2015, when *Scientific American* ran an article by Melinda Moyer headlined, "Why Almost Everything Dean Ornish Says about Nutrition Is Wrong." Like Taubes, Moyer notes that during a time when the prevalence of obesity trebled in the Unites States, Americans dramatically reduced the percentage of calories they consumed from protein and fat while upping the percentage of the carbohydrates that Ornish says we should eat more of. She quotes nutritional epidemiologist Lyn Steffen, who says, "I believe the low-fat message promoted the obesity epidemic." Moyer also berates Ornish for relying on what scientists call "observational studies," which say nothing about cause and effect. People who eat less fat may indeed have fewer heart attacks, but the reason for that could have nothing to do with what they eat—perhaps fat avoiders also exercise more or are less likely to smoke.

In addition, Moyer says, Ornish ignores observational studies with contradictory results, showing that diets high in fat and protein are not associated with heart disease. She faults Ornish for lumping all animal protein together by conflating processed meat products like hot dogs, pepperoni, and sausages with unprocessed meats, when studies show that processed meats are far more harmful than fresh red meat and that there are no problems associated with eating white meat, such as chicken. She also claims that Ornish muddied the water by having his subjects give up smoking and take up stress management and exercise in addition to eating an ultra–low fat diet, suggesting that maybe it was the other factors, not the diet, that benefitted the subjects. "Ornish's arguments against protein and fat are weak, simplistic, and, in a way, irrelevant," she concludes.

Replying to the *Scientific American* editor, Ornish wrote that he wasn't in the habit of responding to ad hominem attacks, but he was making an exception in this case. What followed was a scathing rebuttal that ran nearly four times as long as the original piece. "Her article begins with a gross distortion of what I believe," he wrote. "It's the type of protein, fat, and carbohydrates that matters. The diet I recommend is low in refined carbohydrates and low in harmful fats (including trans fats and some saturated fats) *and* low in animal protein (particularly red meat) but includes beneficial fats (including omega-3 fatty acids), good carbs (including fruits, vegetables, whole grains, legumes, and soy in their natural, unrefined forms), and good proteins (predominantly plant-based)."

Moyer's argument about Americans eating a lower percentage of fat, he said, ignores the fact that we are eating more *total* fat because we're eating more of everything, including refined carbohydrates, which Ornish disapproves of. He said that he cited "several large-scale studies from many different investigators, all of which showed that a diet high in red meat increases the risk of premature death from virtually all causes, even when adjusting for confounding variables. I'm not cherry-picking data; I'm looking at the preponderance of evidence from many studies by leading investigators, such as those at Harvard School of Public Health." Ornish then indulged in an ad hominem attack of his own, berating Moyer for her lack of clinical experience.

"That article came right out of the *National Enquirer* school of journalism," Ornish told me.

Even as the critical blowback intensified, Ornish gained some major allies in his contention that an ultra-low fat diet is the key to heart health. In 1985, Dr. Caldwell B. Esselstyn, a surgeon at the Cleveland Clinic, launched a twelve-year study involving twenty-four patients referred to him by cardiologists at the clinic. The main criteria for inclusion in Esselstyn's program, as was the case in Ornish's early research, was that all participants were suffering from severe coronary artery disease and were beyond the help of surgical procedures such as bypasses and stents. Fifteen had increasing angina. Seven had already undergone bypass surgery. Two had had angioplasty. Four had experienced heart attacks. And three had suffered strokes. They literally had nothing to lose by going on Esselstyn's diet, which had much in common with Ornish's, even though Esselstyn was not aware of Ornish's findings when he launched his own study.

The Cleveland heart patients would follow a plant-based diet containing between 9 and 12 percent of its calories from fat. But "plant-based" was critical. These were Esselstyn's rules as outlined in his 2007 book *Prevent and Reverse Heart Disease*:

→ You may not eat anything with a mother or a face (no meat, poultry, or fish).

→ You cannot eat dairy products.
→ You must not consume oil of any kind—not a drop. (Yes, you devotees of the Mediterranean diet, that includes olive oil.)
→ Generally speaking, you cannot eat nuts or avocados.

By eliminating those dietary offenders and encouraging the consumption of vegetables (except those oily avocados), legumes, whole grains, and fruits—and allowing alcohol in moderation—Esselstyn claimed that his diet did not contain "a single item of any food known to cause or promote the development of vascular disease" and assured participants in his study that if they complied (his italics) "*for the rest of your lives you will never again have to count calories or worry about your weight.*" For added protection, the subjects also took modest doses of a cholesterol-lowering drug.

While Ornish delivered his dietary advice in a mellow, feel-good manner befitting someone who had learned at the feet of a swami, Esselstyn was a harsh schoolmaster. "My nutritional program is strict, and allows no short cuts. I am uncompromising. I am authoritative," he wrote. "*There are no exceptions.* Patients must erase the phrase 'This little bit can't hurt' from their vocabulary and from their thinking. As we have learned, the opposite is true: every little bit *can* hurt—and does." Esselstyn based that assertion on research that showed even a morsel of fat compromises the body's ability to form nitric oxide, a chemical that helps blood to flow smoothly. Plant foods, alternatively, are rich in an amino acid that is essential for the formation of nitric oxide. Unlike Ornish's diet, Esselstyn's plan requires neither meditation nor exercise. He is convinced that diet alone can conquer heart disease and also feels that "every human being has just so many behavior modification units available." If he asked them for too much, patients would be more likely to fail.

CALDWELL B. ESSELSTYN

APPROACH

DIET ALONE PREVENTS AND REVERSES HEART DISEASE

DO THIS

PLANT-BASED FOODS AND
9–12% OF CALORIES FROM FAT

NOT THIS

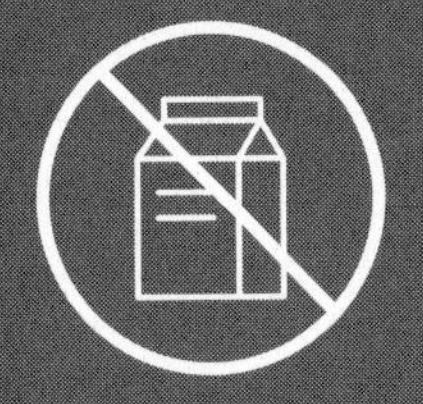

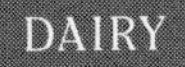

DAIRY

OIL OF ANY KIND

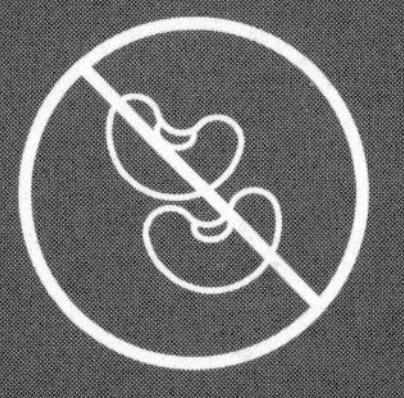

NUTS OR
AVOCADOS

MEAT, POULTRY,
OR FISH

Research that Esselstyn reviewed showed that in parts of the world where heart disease is nearly nonexistent, diets are low in fat, and blood cholesterol levels are consistently below 150 milligrams per deciliter (mg/dL). In rural China, where little animal protein was consumed, the normal range of cholesterol was between 90 and 150 mg/dL. The highlanders of New Guinea, who subsisted on a diet mainly of tubers, experienced no coronary disease. And in the United States, the famous Framingham Heart Study, which has tracked thousands of residents of the city of Framingham, Massachusetts, for decades, found only five instances of people who had maintained a cholesterol level lower than 150 mg/dL but developed coronary artery disease.

Before launching his study, Esselstyn tested his theories on a convenient guinea pig—himself. Although he was fit, having been a member of the U.S. rowing team that won a gold medal in 1952 when he was twenty-one years old, the effects of poor diet could be seen in his family. Every member had died early. His father and father-in-law suffered from diabetes, strokes, coronary artery disease, and cancers of the prostrate, colon, and lung. In April 1985, at age fifty-two, Esselstyn gave up eating meat. By June, his cholesterol had dropped from 185 mg/dL to 155. That wasn't enough for him, so he dropped every source of oil and dairy fat from his diet, and his cholesterol level fell to 119 mg/dL, well below the American average of 215 mg/dL, which is at the extreme high end of the level recommended by the American Heart Association.

By the end of Esselstyn's twelve-year-long study, every one of the subjects, who had begun with an average cholesterol level of 246 mg/dL, had dropped to an average of less than 150. Every angiogram (an X-ray of coronary arteries) taken showed their heart disease had stopped progressing or had been reversed. Angina had been lessened in every member of the group who had suffered from it prior to joining. Exercise capacity had improved. In clear contrast, heart disease had progressed in all six of the original patients who dropped out of the study and resumed their former eating habits. Five had undergone bypasses or angioplasty and two had died from coronary disease.

"*Among the fully compliant patients, during the twelve-year study, there was not one further clinical episode of worsening coronary artery disease,*" Esselstyn wrote (the italics are his). "We can go directly to the bottom line," he continued. "This is it: *if you follow a plant-based nutrition program to reduce your total cholesterol level to below 150 md/dL and the LDL* ["bad" cholesterol] *level to less than 80 mg/dL, you cannot deposit fat in your coronary arteries.* Period."

Research also showed that the benefits of a low-fat, plant-based diet extended to other so-called diseases of affluence—maladies associated with economically developed countries. In addition to heart disease, diabetes and several cancers were lower in areas of the world where people ate very small amounts of animal-derived foods.

Perhaps the most prominent of these studies was the China-Oxford-Cornell Study on Dietary, Lifestyle, and Disease Mortality Characteristics in 65 Rural Chinese Counties, which, mercifully, is usually called simply the China Study. Launched in 1983 and overseen by T. Colin Campbell of Cornell University, the research project spanned two decades and was, at the time, the most comprehensive examination of diet, lifestyle, and disease ever undertaken. The *New York Times* called it the Grand Prix of epidemiology. Campbell alone authored or coauthored 350 scientific articles based on the China work, which he outlined, along with conclusions drawn from many other scientists, in his 2005 bestselling book, *The China Study*.

Key among his findings was that the rural Chinese not only consumed one-third less protein as a percentage of calories in their diets than

Americans but also obtained a minimal amount of their protein from animal sources (about 10 percent), while Americans obtained more than 80 percent of their protein from meat, eggs, and dairy products. As a result:

- → The cholesterol level in the Chinese participants ranged between 70 and 170 ml/dL versus between 200 and 300 ml/dL for Americans.
- → Chinese who ate the most animal-based foods suffered higher rates of coronary disease, cancer, and diabetes.
- → Strikingly, American men were *seventeen times more likely* to die from heart disease than rural Chinese.
- → The Chinese received only 14 percent of their calories from fat on average, versus 36 percent for Americans at that time.
- → The Chinese diet was three times as high in fiber than the American diet.
- → The Chinese actually consumed more calories per pound of body weight than Americans, yet had lower rates of obesity. Among Chinese, participants who were vegan or vegetarian were anywhere from five to thirty pounds slimmer than their compatriots. (Campbell cited research showing that vegetarians had higher rates of metabolism during rest, meaning they burned more calories than carnivores.)

"The message could not be simpler," wrote Campbell. "Eat as many whole fruits, vegetables, and whole grains as you can."

As the years passed, Ornish and his colleagues also showed that the benefits of a low-fat, low-stress lifestyle could extend far beyond cardiac health. In 2005, Ornish partnered with Dr. Peter Carroll, chair of urology

CHINA STUDY STATISTICS

TWO DECADES-LONG COMPARISON STUDY OF THE DIET AND HEALTH RESULTS OF CHINESE PEOPLE IN 65 RURAL COUNTIES AND OF AMERICANS.

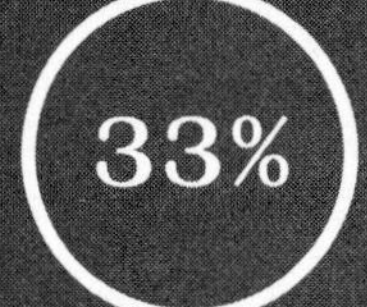

CHINESE PARTICIPANTS CONSUMED 33% LESS PROTEIN AS A PERCENTAGE OF CALORIES.

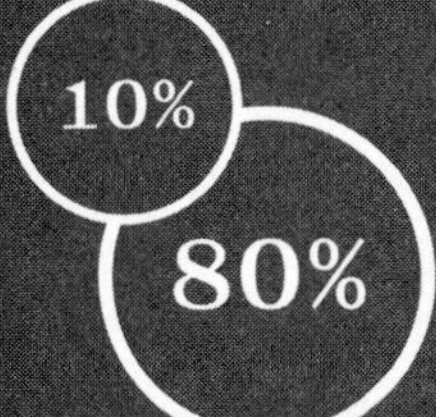

CHINESE PARTICIPANTS GOT 10% OF THEIR PROTEIN FROM ANIMAL SOURCES; AND AMERICAN PARTICIPANTS GOT 80%.

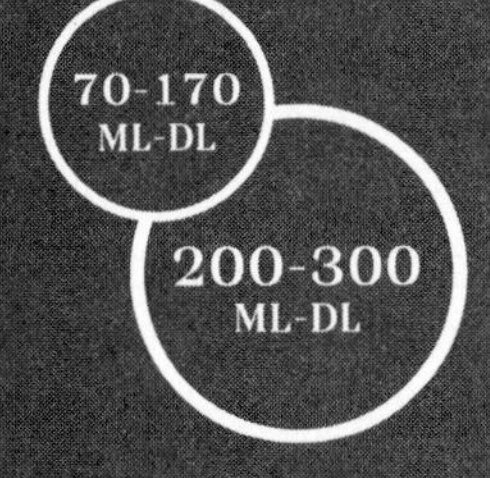

CHINESE PARTICIPANTS' CHOLESTEROL LEVELS RANGED FROM 70 TO 170ML/DL; WHEREAS AMERICAN PARTICIPANTS WERE 200 TO 300ML/DL.

AMERICAN PARTICIPANTS WERE 17X MORE LIKELY TO DIE FROM HEART DISEASE.

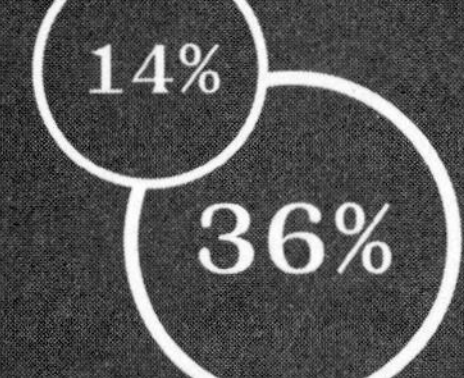

CHINESE PARTICIPANTS CONSUMED 14% OF THEIR CALORIES FROM FAT; AMERICANS CONSUMED 36% OF THEIR CALORIES FROM FAT.

CHINESE PARTICIPANTS CONSUMED 3X MORE FIBER.

at the University of California, San Francisco, and Dr. William Fair, chair of urology and urologic oncology at Memorial Sloan Kettering Cancer Center in Manhattan, to show that the progression of prostate cancer could be stopped and even reversed in patients following the Ornish program. It was the first experimental evidence ever to show that cancer of any type could be beaten if patients made lifestyle changes, and Ornish suspects the same may be true for breast cancer.

Three years later, Ornish and Dr. Elizabeth Blackburn of the University of California, San Francisco, found evidence that his lifestyle regimen could let us all live longer by increasing the length of telomeres, the ends of humans' chromosomes. Longer telomeres lead to longer lives.

Ornish was also able to conduct an angiogram to measure artery plaque in a sixty-year-old male who had followed the Ornish plan since age nineteen. The subject's cholesterol level was 125 mg/dL. He had the clean arteries of a fourteen-year-old boy. The subject's name was Dean Ornish. "It made me happy that I'm a good poster boy for the Dean Ornish program," he told me.

I'm anything but a Dean Ornish poster boy. I confess to a fondness for fatty heritage pork chops and a weakness for grass-fed steaks. When I met with Ornish, I could not recall a day when I hadn't consumed some animal product. I adore good artisanal bread, especially when it's slathered with cultured butter. I have never meditated or practiced yoga in my life and am profoundly skeptical of all things spiritual and remotely New Age–y. But I decided to take Ornish's advice on what to eat. It seemed extreme, but maybe it was a diet I could live with. I decided to give eating the Ornish way a one-week trial just to see if I could do it.

In preparation, I poured over the recipes that Ornish includes in his books. Although my wife and I are both enthusiastic home cooks with a varied repertoire and what I thought was a well-stocked pantry, I immediately realized that for a week of mostly vegan meals our cupboard was woefully bare. Ingredients we lacked included buckwheat soba noodles, quinoa, instant polenta, vegetable stock, tamari sauce, silken tofu, green lentils, garbanzo beans, the nonsugar sweetener Splenda, and Pam cooking spray. I would also have to spend a great deal of time in the produce department to obtain a veritable cornucopia of fruits and vegetables, which might have been fresh and readily available in Ornish's home state of California, but were out of season in March in Vermont, where I live, and worse for the wear from the distance they had traveled. Inside the natural foods store, my cart slowly filled with sweet peppers (both red and green), Anaheim peppers, jalapeños, zucchinis, cucumbers, green beans, snow peas, Chinese cabbages, broccoli, tomatoes (fresh and canned), eggplants, strawberries, kiwifruit, a pineapple, mung bean sprouts, and four different kinds of mushrooms—umami-rich substitutes for meat in many Ornish meals.

I pushed the cart into the labyrinthine bulk foods section of the store to score the necessary beans and grains. It was a section I had rarely ventured into, and I immediately understood why: I lack the patience to search row after row of clear-plastic, cylindrical containers; peer at hand-written labels until I find a canister of what I'm looking for; scrounge around for a little plastic bag; fill it; and scribble a number on the label. To be fair, most of the other patrons, veteran bulk foodies, I assumed, seemed comfortable with the routine and much more efficient than I. After two and a half hours in the market, I had picked up fifty different items amounting to $239 worth of groceries, nearly twice what I would have paid for my typical cart, which would have contained expensive meat and seafood.

Back home, I quickly settled into my new dining routine. Making breakfasts was easy and satisfied my hunger, although I sorely missed pastured eggs, and my meals didn't exactly win rave reviews. My grown daughter visited and commented that the oatmeal with ginger and orange concentrate reminded her of going wilderness camping with me far beyond the reach of electricity and refrigeration. My wife allowed that the oatmeal was "pretty good" and promptly added a glop of butter and a heaping tablespoon of dark brown sugar to her serving. One plate of California eggs (the whites of two eggs, a tomato slice, and a basil leaf on a slice of dry whole-wheat toast) made me realize that, meringues aside, it's yolks that make eggs delicious. Surprisingly, after an entire adulthood of starting every morning with a cup of black coffee, I suffered no symptoms of caffeine withdrawal when, in obedience to Ornish's program, I skipped my daily fix.

Lunches consisted of vegetable stews, bean salads, and lentil salads, all filling and tasty, but requiring far more prep time than I normally allot. However, the midday demands on my time were nothing compared to the hour or two I spent getting dinner on the table each night. That entire cartload of vegetables had to be sliced, diced, chopped, minced, mashed, or julienned before being boiled, steamed, simmered, or braised in vegetable stock, but never (horrors!) sautéed in olive oil. On the upside, my knife skills improved as my week bent over cutting boards progressed. We dined well on black-bean burritos with a faux guacamole made from garlic and fresh peas whirred in the food processor, ratatouille with a bright spicy kick, and roasted Anaheim peppers stuffed with instant polenta, fresh corn kernels, and cilantro served over spicy black beans. Again, the food was filling and surprisingly good—until I prepared a plate of buckwheat noodles. The noodles looked disconcertingly like earthworms. As for taste, let's just say the visuals did not mislead.

The noodle fiasco was an exception. My real issue with eating the Ornish way was the time it took to prepare lunches and dinners. If only we had the services of a personal chef, following the diet would have been a breeze.

From the outset, however, I had rigged the system to my advantage. I chose a week when we had no social engagements and neither of us would be traveling. I preplanned all the meals and shopped in advance for the ingredients we would need. There would be no dashing out at the last minute for a pack of dried black mushrooms. And I picked a week when I could spare the time to do all the cooking.

Fate intervened on day five. Business friends from out of state were staying nearby and on the spur of the moment suggested we go to a restaurant for dinner. Emboldened by the success of four relatively painless, booze-less, low-fat days, I agreed to meet at a small cozy place we frequent. As soon as I stepped into the restaurant with its familiar scents and faces, I understood what an alcoholic must feel like upon stepping into his favorite bar after a month in rehab. The hostess greeted us like old friends and escorted us to our preferred quiet corner table. My companions ordered cocktails. Summoning my willpower, I resisted—for about a second. Neither bourbon nor red vermouth contains fat, or so I rationalized, albeit lamely.

But it was as if the chef had selected the evening's special as a way to test my meat-deprived resolve. I felt my willpower draining away as the waitress described Korean barbecued short ribs from cattle that had been grass fed on a nearby farm. She said the meat was placed over scallion rice and accompanied by Asian slaw and a honey sesame bun. I succumbed. And, of course, I had a couple of glasses of Russian River Zinfandel. And perhaps a spoonful or two—okay, three—of my wife's maple crème brûlée in the spirit of, if you're going to sin, sin big.

Fortunately, I climbed right back on the Ornish bandwagon the next morning with a mushroom and egg white scramble and remained aboard for the rest of the week. My wife claimed that I looked better. My jeans certainly fit better. And the scale showed that, despite my night of debauchery, I'd actually dropped a couple of pounds.

More important, I learned that I could actually follow a low-fat, plant-based diet—if I absolutely had to. But that was a very big if. Complying with the advice of Ornish, Esselstyn, and Campbell would mean giving up a lot of things that bring me tremendous pleasure—a great steak grilled and eaten outside on a summer evening, fall-off-the-bone barbecued ribs, smoked salmon with a dab of crème fraîche, and vibrant artisanal cheese. I don't want to forgo relaxing in a restaurant and instead sit on the edge of my chair summoning every ounce of willpower as I watch my tablemates blissfully chew through foods that are banned from my plate. And then there are those divine eggs from my backyard flock.

Low-fat advocates make a convincing scientific case, but, like the puritanical preacher Sylvester Graham, they play down or completely ignore the important, sensual role that food plays in our aesthetic and cultural life—something that means a lot to me. Was there a better way?

CHAPTER SIX

LOW-CARB COUNTRY

Dr. Arthur Agatston likes to describe himself as an "accidental diet doctor." Some accident.

True, Agatston has spent the bulk of his career as a cardiologist with offices in the South Beach district of Miami Beach. He regularly sees patients in his private practice, and he also conducts research as a professor at the Miller School of Medicine, at the University of Miami. Agatston's work resulted in numerous scientific papers, making him highly respected in his field of expertise, but unknown beyond.

His specialty is noninvasive cardiac imaging—using technologies such as computerized tomography (CT) to look at the heart and the surrounding blood vessels without resorting to surgery. His first claim to fame came in 1990, when he developed ways of measuring calcium levels in coronary arteries.

Calcium is one of the components of arterial plaque, and high levels indicate a risk for heart attacks, similar to high levels of cholesterol and elevated blood pressure. The Agatston score and Agatston method, as they are known by heart specialists, are commonly used by doctors today. Tests to determine the score are inexpensive and take very little time. Agatston half-jokingly says that a doctor's failure to give the test to patients who might have heart disease should constitute medical malpractice. I wondered why Doctor Dennis had never had me tested for arterial calcium and made a mental note to bring up the question at my next physical exam.

To help his obese patients at his cardiac practice lose weight, Agatston, who freely admits that, like most physicians, he originally knew very little about nutrition, dutifully suggested that they follow the American Heart Association's recommendations to eat a low-fat, high-carbohydrate diet, which he also followed. But he noticed that even those who stayed religiously within the association's guidelines kept getting fatter, and their blood chemistries continued to worsen.

Agatston almost gave up recommending that people who came to him go on diets, relying instead on drugs, like statins, to control their blood cholesterol and diuretics to lower their blood pressure. But in 1995, after reviewing scientific literature on weight loss, he concluded that fats were not the cause of obesity and related heart disease. Instead, the culprits were carbohydrates, specifically simple carbohydrates such as those in sugars, highly processed snack foods, and white flour.

With that in mind, he developed an eating plan he called the Modified Carbohydrate Diet, which he printed up and handed out to his patients. As they saw pounds fall off and waistlines narrow, they shared photocopies of Agatston's plan with friends. A local television station publicized the program. Agatston got a book deal. Someone—Agatston thought it was he, his wife claimed it was she, and he admits that she was probably right—insisted the program needed a catchier name than the Modified Carbohydrate Diet. He rechristened it the South Beach Diet.

Published in 2003, the resulting book became an instant *New York Times* bestseller and remained one for four years. It, and a dozen or so spin-offs authored by Agatston, have sold nearly twenty-five million copies in both English and Spanish. Bette Midler and the president of the American Heart Association both went on the diet. Agatston appeared regularly on national television and was the subject of numerous magazine profiles. In 2015, Nutrisystem, Inc., a $700 million weight-loss company primarily known for its food delivery program, bought the rights to the South Beach Diet for $15 million. The accidental diet doctor had become a celebrity diet doctor, and a wealthy one at that.

Yet when I met with Agatston on a gorgeous March afternoon at his offices, which are still in South Beach, I could detect no trappings of celebrity. He still sees a regular stream of patients through what is called a concierge practice, where patients pay him an annual retainer of roughly $12,000 per family, with no restrictions on how often they visit and how long their appointments last. For Agatston, it means that he can see a few patients a day for longer periods and still find time to conduct scientific research. It also allows him to focus on prevention.

"I love seeing patients, but I like to see just a few a day," he told me. "Otherwise I would have a full waiting room and be seeing thirty patients a day and then spending most of my time filling out documents for insurance companies and Medicare."

Agatston and I were among the very few decidedly unhip old white guys clad in faded khaki trousers and Oxford shirts in that part of town, where the natives favored designer leisure wear; multiple body piercings; eye-catching hairstyles in vibrant colors; and elaborate, plentiful tattoos. Agatston was much younger looking than his seventy-plus years and carried himself like a bantamweight boxer (boxing being one of his regular athletic pursuits, along with tennis and golf). True to his word, the waiting room at the Agatston Center for Private Medicine was empty when I arrived. With its comfy leatherette armchairs and dark wood flooring, it looked more like the lobby of a pricey hotel than the waiting room of any doctor's office I'd ever sat in, thumbing wrinkled, months-old issues of popular magazines.

Were it not for an assortment of plastic reproductions of human hearts and artificial cross sections of blood vessels, Agatston's own office could have been the work space of any successful executive, albeit one who was tie-less and worked from behind a stand-up desk, which he claims is beneficial to his overall well-being and prevents him from succumbing to the dreaded "sitting disease." He spoke rapidly, in a voice that still betrayed his Long Island roots four decades after he graduated from New York University's medical school. And like many academics, he frequently illustrated his points by opening an at-the-ready library of PowerPoint presentations.

In formulating the South Beach Diet in the late 1990s, Agatston focused on cardiac studies related to something called the insulin resistance syndrome, which interfered with the body's ability to properly process glucose as fuel. His research showed that the carbohydrates we eat are broken down into glucose. But glucose, also called blood sugar, cannot be absorbed by the body's cells on its own. That requires insulin, a hormone excreted by the pancreas.

Complex carbohydrates, like those found in leafy green vegetables, break down slowly. Insulin goes about its work at a leisurely pace, and blood sugar rises and then falls gradually, leaving the eater with a sense of fullness. But simple carbohydrates break down rapidly. Blood sugar spikes. To deal with the rush, insulin floods the system, making blood sugar levels plummet, causing cravings for more food. A quick carbohydrate fix soothes those cravings, but ultimately packs on pounds.

Agatston also noticed that until the twentieth century, coronary thrombosis (which happens when a clot blocks blood supply to the heart) was virtually unreported in the medical literature. Even though Americans consumed large quantities of meat and dairy, they apparently were not dying in great numbers from heart attacks. But by the 1950s, cardiac arrests had become epidemic, causing 50 percent of all deaths. Agatston blamed the sudden surge on an increase in the consumption of simple carbohydrates and artificial trans fats (which are manufactured by adding hydrogen to liquid vegetable oils to make them solid and were once commonly used in processed foods).

He also studied the effects of dietary fiber, which slows the absorption of sugar, resulting in less dramatic swings in blood sugar levels and fewer cravings. Processing removes fiber from foods. A glass of processed apple juice, for instance, contains virtually no fiber, but the apples that go into making it contain twelve grams or more of fiber, nearly half of the recommended daily requirement for adults, according to the American Heart Association. A cup of white flour delivers less than four grams of fiber, but 100 percent whole-wheat flour has four times that amount.

Being a cardiologist, Agatston was leery about the effects of eating large quantities of saturated fats—the type found in red meat and dairy products. True, you could lose weight and still consume saturated fats, as long as you avoided simple carbohydrates, as demonstrated by Robert Atkins in the early 1970s and by the corpulent William Banting more than a century earlier. But Agatston felt that even as the pounds disappeared, eating saturated fat could negatively affect your blood chemistry and leave you more vulnerable to heart attack and stroke.

The South Beach Diet takes all these observations into account. The diet encourages participants to eat what Agatston calls "good carbohydrates" and "good fats," such as those found in nutrient-dense and fiber-heavy unprocessed vegetables and grains. He also encourages the consumption of lean red meat, poultry, olive oil, and nuts. Like fiber, fat and protein help slow the absorption of carbohydrates. "All the data now show that good fats are good for you," Agatston told me. "Avoiding them on an extreme low-fat diet is less healthful than consuming them."

According to the gospel of Arthur Agatston, a slice of supermarket white bread is akin to poison. He says that it is not only stripped of nutrients but also more fattening and worse for your health than ice cream or a spoonful of pure table sugar. A glass of orange juice from a carton has about the same effect on your health as a can of soda, yet a whole orange is fine because its high fiber content slows down your body's absorption of the sugars it contains. Wine in moderation is permissible, but water, of course, is the very best thing you can drink. The worst—here comes bad news for all lovers of microbrews—is beer, whose maltodextrin sugars, he says, are more fattening than table sugar, lending scientific validity for the term *beer belly*.

All that remained was for Agatston to test his dietary theories on an appropriate guinea pig. Fortunately, a middle-aged man with a growing paunch was readily available—Agatston himself. He followed his own advice for a week, and lost nearly eight pounds.

Because of his emphasis on eating "good" carbs and avoiding fatty meats and dairy products, Agatston bristles when South Beach is lumped together with the low-carb, high-protein-and-fat diet fads that have swept the country and place no restrictions on the amount and types of fat consumed. The most notable among those is the program put forward in *Dr. Atkins' Diet Revolution*. First published in 1972, the book and its spinoffs went on to sell more than 15 million copies and made Atkins a household name. It's easy to understand why Agatston would disapprove of comparisons with Robert Atkins. In the Atkins world, there are no good or bad carbohydrates, just bad ones. Early in the book, Atkins proclaims, "This diet is an anti-carbohydrate diet." He describes carbohydrates as "poison" and follows that by declaring "carbohydrate poisoning" is the cause of the most chronic diseases of the twentieth century. True, he allows salads of leafy greens during the initial phase of his diet, which provide the only carbohydrates that can be eaten during that stage. But Atkins only permits this indulgence because simple green salads are so low in carbs that they have the same effect as cutting out carbohydrates altogether.

In later phases of the diet, Atkins allows the reintroduction of more carbohydrates, mainly through leafy greens, summer squash, string beans, tomatoes, onions, and other nonstarchy plant-based fare. Among the foods that Atkins considered toxic and forever banished are bread, crackers, milk, flour, bananas, corn, potatoes, peas, and dried beans. Orange juice is another. Why drink it, Atkins says, when you can get all the benefits and none of the sugar by taking a vitamin C pill? Alcohol is banned in the early stages of the diet and frowned upon in the later ones. Atkins claims that booze affects the body in the same ways as carbohydrates and is the number-one problem for weight control among many of his cocktail-loving patients. He takes pride that not a single recipe in his book contains more than 6 grams of carbohydrate per serving and recommends that those following his plan consume no more than 40 grams of carbohydrates per day. The U.S. Dietary Guidelines say that an average woman should be getting between 225 and 325 grams.

Atkins places no limits whatsoever on how much protein and fat his patients consume, claiming that followers "have lost weight on bacon and eggs for breakfast, on heavy cream in their coffee, on mayonnaise in their salads, butter sauce on their lobster; on spareribs, roast duck, pastrami; on my special cheesecake for dessert." He approves of slathering mayonnaise on cold salmon and recommends butter on asparagus and Roquefort dressing for green salads. And feel free to have any cheese as a snack.

His bacon and cheese soufflé contains ½ cup of butter, 1½ cups of heavy cream, 2 cups of shredded cheddar cheese, 8 eggs, and ½ cup of crumbled bacon. In addition to ground beef, an Atkins bacon cheeseburger calls for bacon and cheddar cheese—and it's fried in bacon fat. His cottage cheese and sour cream salad is dressed with 2 cups of cottage cheese and 1 cup of sour cream. And the cheesecake he is so proud of is full of heavy cream, whipped cream cheese, and eggs, but it is made with a sugar-free saccharin-based sweetener, because sugar is taboo.

Main courses are no problem for Atkins. "A patient christened it the steak-and-salad diet—and that does rather sum up the plot of it," Atkins wrote in *Dr. Atkins' Diet Revolution*, proceeding to say that you can replace the steak with "almost any kind of meat, fish, or fowl! . . . including such usually forbidden goodies as ham, spareribs, bacon, roast beef, corned beef, roast duckling, lobster with butter sauce."

Atkins claimed that his patients' blood chemistry improved even as they gobbled all of those supposedly unhealthy foods. One participant

SOUTH BEACH DIET

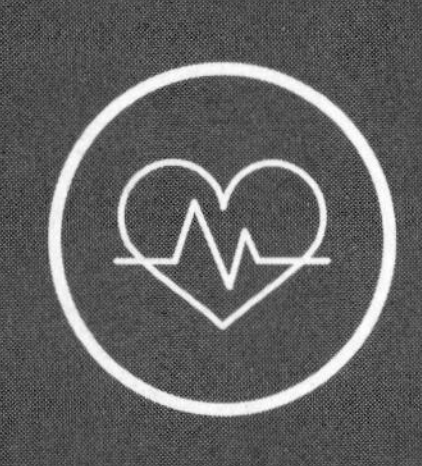

ARTHUR AGATSTON

CARDIOLOGIST AND CREATOR OF THE SOUTH BEACH DIET

ALLOWED

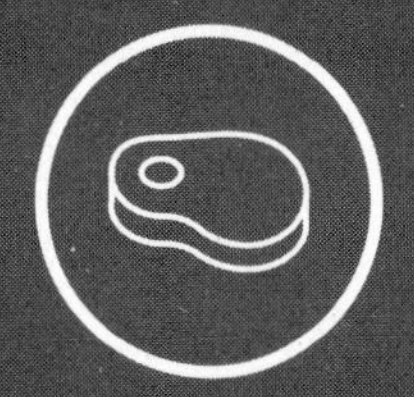

UNLIMITED PROTEIN AND FAT

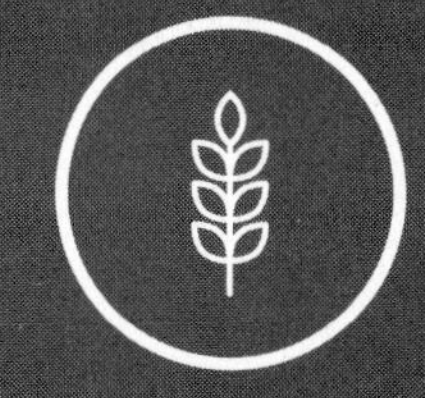

WHOLE GRAINS

SOME FRUIT

NOT ALLOWED

SIMPLE CARBOHYDRATES

SUGAR

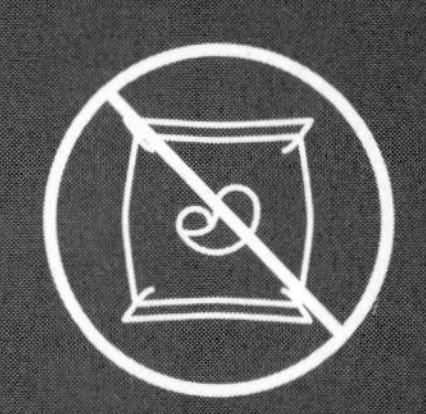

PROCESSED SNACK FOODS

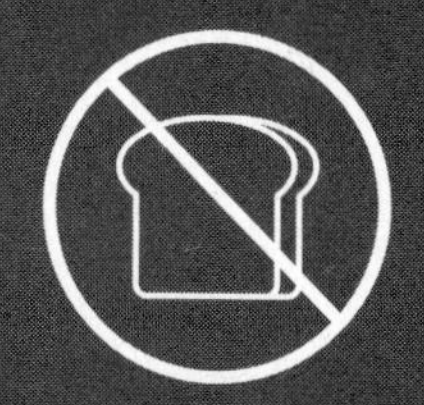

WHITE FLOUR

RELATED TO

KETO

ATKINS' DIET

PALEO

routinely had a two-egg cheese omelet washed down with coffee with heavy cream for breakfast. Lunch was a huge steak and lettuce salad with blue-cheese dressing. For dinner, he ate more steak and perhaps a green vegetable. The guy lost twenty pounds in two months and, says Atkins, his triglyceride and cholesterol levels tumbled.

I was surprised to find scientific validation for some of Atkins' stances. In a 2003 study of fifty-three obese women, Bonnie Brehm, of the University of Cincinnati, reported that those on a low-carbohydrate diet, such as Atkins', lost nineteen pounds over six months, more than twice the eight and a half pounds lost by the similarly chubby cohort on a low-fat regime. Blood pressure, blood chemistry, and blood sugar content improved for both groups. The take-home message was that during a six-month-long experiment, women could lose more weight on a low-carb diet than those on a low-fat plan, without increasing their risk of a heart attack. But the experiment ended after six months, which in the world of nutrition studies is brief.

A subsequent study by Alain Nordmann of the University Hospital in Basel, Switzerland, tracked more subjects, some on a low-carb diet and others on a low-fat diet, over a year. For the first six months, the results mirrored those of the Cincinnati study. At the end of the year, however, both groups had lost equal amounts of weight. And although the high-fat participants had more favorable levels of triglycerides and HDL cholesterol (so-called good cholesterol), the high-carb contingent had lower levels of LDL cholesterol (the bad kind). In plain terms, the results were a wash. Participants on both diets lost the same amount of weight and improved their blood cholesterol levels, though in different ways.

Science suggests that perhaps you can harmlessly lose a few quick pounds by dining on beef and butter and avoiding grains and starchy vegetables—over the short term. But studies that take the long view have nothing but bad news about the health consequences for low-carb devotees. Polish nutritionist Maciej Banach looked at ten years of data compiled between 1999 and 2010 on nearly 25,000 participants in the CDC's National Health and Nutrition Examination Survey conducted in the United States. He found that those who consumed low-carb diets had a 32 percent higher chance of dying from all causes than those with the highest carbohydrate consumption, and a 51 percent greater chance of dying from cardiovascular disease. "Low-carbohydrate diets might be useful in the short term to lose weight, lower blood pressure, and improve blood glucose control," Banach wrote, "but our study suggests that in the long term they are linked with an increased risk of death from any cause, and deaths due to cardiovascular disease, cerebrovascular disease [stroke], and cancer."

Alas, Atkins' final years proved to be a poor recommendation to do as he said. Standing six feet tall and weighing 258 pounds, he qualified as clinically obese. He suffered a heart attack in 2002 at age seventy-one (which he claimed was not caused by following his diet) and died a year later from head injuries suffered after a fall on an icy sidewalk outside his Manhattan offices. Although family members deny it, rumors persist that heart problems led to his fatal tumble. Three years after the doctor's death, his company, Atkins Nutritionals, filed for bankruptcy.

Today, nearly five decades after he published *Dr. Atkins' Diet Revolution,* Atkins' legacy remains alive and well. Almost offhandedly in the first pages of his book he wrote, "As cavemen, we humans evolved mainly on a diet of meat. And that's what our bodies were and are built to handle. For fifty million years our bodies had to deal with only minute amounts of carbohydrates—and unrefined carbohydrates, at that."

It took thirteen years for the term *paleo* to fully enter the nutritional mainstream. Unusual in the world of fad diets (its proponents would tell you that it is a fad that has lasted for hundreds of thousands of years or more), the concept that the foods consumed by our prehistoric ancestors are those that to this day provide humans with optimal nutrition was introduced in one of the world's most highly respected scientific journals. In 1985, Dr. S. Boyd Eaton, a medical professor at Atlanta's Emory University, published an article in the *New England Journal of Medicine* entitled "Paleolithic Nutrition—A Consideration of Its Nature and Current Implications." Three years later, Eaton fleshed out (so to speak) his theories in a book called *The Paleolithic Prescription*. Hundreds of megaselling paleo books followed, including prominent titles like Loren Cordain's *The Paleo Diet*, Robb Wolf's *The Paleo Solution*, and Diane Sanfilippo's *Practical Paleo*, along with a host of books affixing "paleo" to almost every culinary tradition imaginable: paleo Latin American, paleo Korean, paleo Chinese, paleo Mediterranean, and, for those cooks who appreciate a touch of anachronistic irony, "paleo" Instant Pot recipes.

Eaton, now in his early eighties, is a white-haired patrician New Englander (he grew up in Maine but lives in Georgia). Like Agatston, he came to nutrition by a roundabout route. He graduated from Harvard Medical School, where he specialized in radiology of muscles and bones. During his tenure at Emory, a good number of his patients played for the Atlanta Braves baseball team and the Atlanta Falcons football team. The founding principle of his dietary work is that organisms function best when they operate under conditions originally selected by evolution. When modern humans evolved, we were all hunters and gatherers. That lasted until the advent of agriculture, only 10,000 years ago—far too recently, Eaton contends, to permit our bodies to evolve to handle the novel foods that were either scarce or nonexistent before the invention of farming, most noticeably the abundance of carbohydrates brought about by the domestication of wheat, barley, and other grains. According to Eaton, "We are genetic Stone Agers."

As such, we should emphasize lean meats in our diet, like those produced by wild game. Real Stone Agers ate three times the amount of protein as modern humans, according to Eaton. "We have an innate desire for meat. It's literally in our genes," he told a conference of prominent nutritionists in 2015, pointing out that meat is the preferred food for the remaining hunter-gatherer societies around the world. During the Paleolithic Age, humans also ate three times more fruits, roots, and seeds than we do now, in the process consuming between five and ten times as much fiber.

"We traditionally divide our foods into four basic groups," Eaton writes in *The Paleolithic Prescription*, "(1) meat and fish, (2) vegetables and fruit, (3) milk and milk products, and (4) breads and cereals. Yet before agriculture, people derived their nutrients from just the first two groups."

In Eaton's view, by deviating from the diet we were designed to consume, humans have brought a scourge of ailments upon themselves that our cave-dwelling ancestors never experienced. These include chronic conditions such as atherosclerosis, or hardening of the arteries (which leads to heart attack and stroke); high blood pressure; diabetes; cancer; osteoporosis; tooth decay; and the epidemic of obesity. Eaton categorizes these as "diseases of civilization." He observes that before the first human planted a seed or raised a sheep, these diseases simply did not exist, or were extremely rare.

Some critics argue that early humans were free of these diseases because they simply didn't live long enough to suffer their effects. Eaton responds that while it is true that paleo folks had short average life expectancies (about thirty-five years), it was because of high levels of mortality among infants and children. Once early humans had cleared those hurdles, they could expect to live to the age of sixty or beyond, plenty of time to develop heart problems, cancer, and diabetes. Skeletal remains indicate that they were as tall or taller than modern humans and in tremendous physical shape—as strong as today's elite athletes, according to Eaton.

He recognizes that no modern human is going to spear a woolly mammoth or spend hours scratching the ground for roots, but he offers a "Paleolithic prescription" for how today's shoppers can get many of the benefits of his diet in a modern grocery store. (One of his favorites among the countless cartoons spoofing his research is one in the *Atlanta Journal-Constitution* portraying a caveman pushing a supermarket cart.)

Complex carbohydrates found in fruits, vegetables, and whole grains should provide 60 percent of calories. The simple carbs of sugar and refined grains are to be avoided. Protein from low-fat sources, like poultry and lean meat, should account for an additional 20 percent of calories. Fat—with the exception of butter, lard, coconut, and palm-derived fats—makes up the remaining 20 percent, provided you consume more unsaturated (liquid at room temperature) than saturated fat (solid at room temperature). Getting enough fiber is important. Fiber supplied by fruits, whole grains, and vegetables can be supplemented with oat or wheat bran. He recommends that modern Paleo dieters take supplements to make sure they are getting the recommended daily levels of vitamins and minerals. Finally—very important—salt intake must be drastically reduced. Cave folk had access to minimal amounts.

Because our nomadic ancestors had yet to invent the ritual of unwinding with a beer or highball, Eaton adds one other stern admonition to his Paleolithic prescription: "abstinence or at least scrupulous restraint in the use of alcohol is . . . most in keeping with our basic biology."

Loren Cordain, a professor at Colorado State University and author of the bestselling *Paleo Diet*, summarizes the diet with six simple rules.

Consume

1. All the lean meats, fish, and seafood you can eat
2. All the fruits and nonstarchy vegetables you can eat
3. No cereals
4. No legumes
5. No dairy products
6. No processed foods

In a Darwinian way, it's easy to find Eaton's theories intellectually satisfying. True, humans have eaten a diet based on only agricultural products for a blink of the evolutionary eye. As Eaton points out, "Put another way, 100,000 generations of humans have been hunters and gatherers; 500 generations have been agriculturalists; 10 have lived in the industrial age." Isn't it logical, then, to conclude that we are genetically designed to eat the way our distant ancestors did?

Some anthropologists claim that there is one big problem with Eaton's theory: it's bunk. The paleo diet "has no basis in archaeological reality," according to Christina Warinner, a professor of anthropology at Harvard, who has done extensive research on the fossilized teeth of hunter-gatherers. In contrast to Eaton's contention that Paleolithic humans ate only fruits, vegetables, and large amounts of lean meat, Warinner found that their diet included large quantities of legumes, tubers, and grains. She notes that humans have no physical adaptations for meat consumption. Our molars are designed to crush plant foods, but we lack the sharp, pointy carnassial teeth that carnivorous animals use to shear and shred meat. She claims that fossil evidence that hunter-gatherers ate huge amounts of meat is the result of animal remains such as bones being more likely than plants to be preserved as fossils. Finally, she says that paleo humans were the original locavores. They subsisted on a wide variety of foods, depending on what was available. There were many, many different paleo diets.

In any case, Marlene Zuk, a professor of ecology, evolution, and behavior at the University of Minnesota and author of the book *Paleofantasy*, asserts that we are not necessarily still stuck with the genes that served ancient humans so well. "We cannot assume that evolution has stopped for humans or that it can take place only ploddingly with tiny steps over hundreds of thousands of years," she writes. "To think of ourselves as misfits in our own time and of our own making flatly contradicts what we now understand about the way evolution works—namely rate matters. That evolution can be fast, slow, or in-between, and that understanding of what makes the difference is far more enlightening, and exciting, than holding our flabby selves up against a vision—accurate or not—of our well-muscled and harmoniously adapted ancestors."

As the human population exploded exponentially after the invention of farming, so, too, did the opportunities for genetic mutations to occur that could better adapt us to changing conditions. With more humans (and therefore more human genes) to work with, a mutation that once would have occurred every 100,000 years in a small population might now happen every 400 years. Some of these mutations are familiar. Our paleo relatives lacked the ability to digest milk after infancy. The gene that allows some of us to do so now evolved over the last 5,000 to 7,000 years, according to Zuk. Similarly, modern societies that consume high levels of carbohydrates have evolved genes that produce amylase, an enzyme that breaks down starches, making them easier for the body to absorb. A gene that helps lower glucose levels in the blood, raised by consumption of carbohydrates, began spreading in the human population at about the same time hunter-gatherers switched over to farming grains.

Ultimately, even if the paleo diet *is* the panacea its advocates claim, it is impossible to adhere to anything close to what our hunter-gather ancestors ate, unless you capture or shoot all the meat you eat and survive off foraging edible wild plants. Flesh from domestic animals is 25 to 30 percent fat, versus a little over an average of 4 percent for that of wild animals. Even the low-fat animal proteins recommended for paleo followers, like skinless turkey breast, have more than twice the fat contained in wild meat. Over the same time, plant breeders have developed varieties of vegetables and fruits that bear no resemblance to those that preagricultural peoples would have dined on. Wild avocadoes are mostly seed and about the size of an olive. Such seemingly different crops as cabbage, broccoli, cauliflower, Brussels sprouts, collard, kale, and kohlrabi are all varieties of a single species, *Brassica oleracea*, a three- to six-foot-tall plant with sprays of tiny yellow flowers that grows on seaside cliffs in Europe. Corn was a grass from Mexico that bore just a few kernels on each plant. Anyone who has seen a weedy Queen Anne's lace plant by a roadside will recognize the closest thing that paleo diners had to our carrots.

Atkins can also take credit for initiating the keto-diet craze. Keto diets are based on the premise that when your body runs out of glucose, its preferred fuel, it starts breaking down fat reserves into molecules called ketones (the *keto* in keto diets), which it can also burn for fuel, a state called ketosis. In his seminal book, Atkins described a hypothetical follower of his diet: "Now for carbohydrate-intolerant Mr. Fat to be in ketosis deliberately is a signal for rejoicing. It is a sign that the unwanted fat is being burned up as fuel. It is a sign of progress toward health, slimness, a stabilized blood sugar, lower triglyceride levels . . . everything else his heart desires—literally and figuratively."

Think of a keto diet as one that a tribe of our Stone Age counterparts might have adopted immediately after killing a buffalo. With no need to forage for sustenance, they could gorge themselves on the unfortunate creature to the exclusion of almost all plant matter. In their modern incarnation, keto diets call for between 60 and 80 percent of calorie intake to come from fat (the USDA recommends 20 to 35 percent), and as little as 5 percent from carbohydrates (versus the USDA's recommendation of between 45 and 65 percent).

"When we're talking about eating keto, we're talking about eating fat. Like, a lot of fat. Probably more than you've ever dreamed of eating, and then about 10 percent more than that," writes Leanne Vogel, author of *The Keto Diet*. She provides a detailed graphic chart on how to add more fat to otherwise lean foods: Toss some bacon into a bowl of salad greens, then dress them with the leftover pan grease, which can also be used to roast vegetables. Scramble eggs with "epic amounts" of coconut oil, a dish made even better if you use only egg yolks (which contain nearly all of an egg's fat). Sauté everything in tallow, lard, duck fat, or, of course, bacon grease.

Keto diets actually work—if your goal is limited to short-term weight loss, and you are not too concerned with your overall heath. A paper in the journal *Nutrients,* by Christophe Kosinski of Lausanne University, in Switzerland, which examined the results of numerous studies on the effects of keto diets, concluded that the preponderance of evidence showed that subjects did lose more weight on high-fat diets than comparable groups assigned high-carbohydrate diets, although the scientists said that there was not enough evidence to prove that the loss would last over time. Counterintuitively, given that fat is generally viewed as Public Enemy Number One when it comes to heart-damaging levels of cholesterol and triglycerides in the blood, the paper found that keto diets reduced levels of total cholesterol—particularly LDL, the "bad" kind—and triglycerides. The study did sound one important note of caution: The *source* of fat in keto diets was critical to healthful outcomes. Participants who got their fat through animal products were twice as likely to develop type 2 diabetes as those on traditional diets. Conversely, keto dieters who took in most of their fat through plant sources were at decreased risk. Ultimately, Kosinski and his associates concluded that more studies were needed "to better assess the long-term use of keto diets on metabolic diseases [like diabetes] and cardiovascular risk factors."

Keto also brings a host of unpleasant side effects. When they first adopt the diet, many people experience "keto flu." As the name implies, the symptoms include headaches, nausea, and diarrhea. Other issues include constipation, dandruff, hair loss, and what Vogel describes as "dragon breath" and body odor. One reason for that rapid weight loss is that you excrete more water when you are in ketosis. As soon as you return to carbs, that water is rapidly replaced, and your weight goes up along with it.

Not wanting to asphyxiate my spouse and close associates with dragon breath, and ever mindful of Doctor Dennis's admonitions not to do anything crazy, I decided to limit my adventures in Low-Carb Country to Agatston's relatively moderate South Beach Diet. Like many diets, Agatston's plan proceeds through a set of decreasingly restrictive phases. His Phase One, which Agatston describes as a kick start, lasts for two weeks and bans bread, rice, potatoes, pasta, sweets, alcohol, and even fruit. Phases Two and Three still limit simple carbs and sugars, but are more lenient. You are allowed to reintroduce fruits, whole-grain bread, brown rice, whole-wheat pasta, and sweet potatoes into your diet, along with small amounts of wine—provided you maintain your desired weight. Should the pounds start returning, it's back to Phase One for you.

When I mentioned to a friend that I intended to embark on the South Beach regime, she rolled her eyes and said, "My husband and I have been on that diet for years. We call it the Chop-Chop Diet." Within two days, I understood exactly what she meant. Even Ornish's program, which vastly improved my knife skills, was nothing to Agatston's. I'd go so far as to say that the first step in eating the South Beach way is to go out and have your favorite chef's knife professionally sharpened and then keep a steel within easy reach every time you deploy it.

One lunch consisted of South Beach Chopped Salad with Tuna—at least I had fair warning with the word *chopped* in the title. The recipe called for me to chop a cucumber, tomato, avocado, some celery, radishes, and (my wrist was getting tired by this point, as was my patience—it was a workday lunch!) romaine lettuce. Oh, yes. I also added a can of tuna. My midafternoon snack called for me to chop more celery. Dinner had me chopping eggplant, cucumbers, cherry tomatoes, and bell peppers, which I added both to the main vegetable course with the eggplant and to the tossed salad. Be forewarned, you'll be eating more bell peppers on South Beach than you ever thought possible. One morning found me fresh out of bed chopping asparagus, mushrooms, and reduced-fat mozzarella cheese for my omelet. Agatston told me that the reward for all this chopping was that my diet would contain enormous quantities of healthful fiber, which slows the digestion of carbohydrates. As a bonus, the beneficial bacteria that live in our intestines feast on the fiber that we are unable to digest. When I jokingly suggested that he should have named his program the High-Fiber Diet, he said, "I'll take that."

Agatston also introduced me to a host of foods that I had steadfastly avoided previously: liquid egg substitute, low-fat mozzarella cheese, foil-wrapped wedges of low-fat Laughing Cow cheese, and low-fat cottage cheese—all of which were unsatisfying substitutes for their genuine counterparts. Since Agatston first introduced the South Beach diet, he has become more lenient—whole eggs have his blessing, as do full-fat dairy products.

Despite being resentful of all that time spent chopping—especially on days when I was busy with work and in a rush to get something, *anything*, on the table—adhering to South Beach created only minor problems. I couldn't grab a wrap or sandwich while rushing through airports. Nor could I find acceptable sustenance amid the offerings of service-station delis. And on occasion, I pined for the days when I used to slap a piece of meat between two slices of bread along with mayonnaise or Dijon mustard and call that lunch.

If Agatston is an accidental diet doctor, he is also an accidental, accidental gluten-free diet doctor. I hadn't thought of it until I met with him, but the strictest part of his carb-restricted diet allows no foods containing wheat, barley, or rye, which all contain the protein gluten. For people who genuinely suffer from celiac disease (about 1 percent of us), ingesting gluten, which damages their small intestine, can lead to chronic fatigue, rashes, severe cramping, osteoporosis, and even death. You know when you truly have the disease. But Agatston is convinced that many people who do not suffer from full-blown celiac disease are still to varying degrees gluten sensitive. Many of these "silent celiacs," as he calls them, don't realize it, even though the protein can afflict them with stomachaches, diarrhea, heartburn, body aches, headaches, fatigue, psoriasis, and rheumatoid arthritis.

I personally know one of these sufferers. My friend Mark Smith, who is the husband of culinary instructor and cookbook author Molly Stevens, just hadn't felt right for as long as he can remember and had accepted that as a normal part of growing older—until his wife went on a book tour. Left alone, he abandoned their usual varied fare and reverted to a bachelor diet heavy on pizza and beer, both of which contain gluten. By the time his wife returned, he was in so much pain that he could barely rise from bed. When the doctor determined that he was gluten sensitive, he and his wife took it a little personally. "We never thought we were *that* type of people," she told me, in jest. But when her husband gave up gluten, his health returned and that meh cloud he'd lived under for so long lifted.

Because Agatston found that many of his patients were gluten sensitive without knowing it and experienced relief during Phase One of his diet, he suggests that everyone should go gluten free, if for no other reason than to make sure they are not silent celiacs. And there's no downside. My South Beach stint showed me that I handled gluten just fine. Alas, that didn't give me permission to indulge in pizza and beer.

Overall, I found South Beach a diet I could live with—but not love. During the cold months of my South Beach stint, I sorely missed our weekly dinners of spaghetti topped with a simple sauce made from tomatoes grown in our garden and frozen in meal-sized portions, enabling us to get a blast of summer brightness on the table in fewer than fifteen minutes during the darkest time of a New England winter. And thank God I'm not afflicted with cravings for cakes, cookies, ice cream, and other desserts. Ideally, I thought, I wanted a diet that did not ban entire food groups, be they fat or carbohydrates, and still allowed me to lose weight.

Such a diet exists.

CHAPTER SEVEN

LOSERS PAY

Just before noon on a summery, late September day, I drove to a run-of-the-mill suburban strip mall, surrendered my credit card, and stepped on the platform of an electronic scale substantial enough to weigh a horse. A vivacious woman with a name tag bearing two pieces of information—her name was Roseanne and she had lost twenty-two pounds in 2002—cheerfully deducted $54.95 from the card, peeled off a pink name tag for me to stick on my shirt, and presented me with a small booklet entitled, Success Story. On the appropriate page, Roseanne affixed a sticker printed out by the scale. It bore the date, my name, and my weight, a near-record high of 236 pounds. I'd regained nearly every ounce I had lost on the diets I'd tried previously. My serial failures added a timely element to my joining WW International, known as Weight Watchers for the first five decades of its existence.

Roseanne invited me to take a seat in a lecture room hidden directly behind the weigh-in booths, saying that the meeting would begin shortly. On the way there, I passed a display of products sold under the WW International brand. It was a gauntlet of tempting goodies. I could "fall in love with flavor" by indulging in chocolate fudge or mocha latte ice cream bars, coconut-chocolate candy bars, mint patties, pasta, English toffee, or jalapeño string cheese. I could also pick up one of the organization's cookbooks or the latest issue of its magazine, and—my favorite—a set of portion-control wineglasses, which, in retrospect, I should have bought. I did take home a box of frozen chocolate fudge bars and a pack of string cheese. I found nothing to love about the frozen bars, which had a cardboard flavor. The string cheese tasted exactly like run-of-the-mill string cheese and was slightly lower in calories than the store brand I had in my fridge (left over from my South Beach days), but it cost twice as much.

The room itself would be familiar to anyone who has spent time in a college class. Three rows of chairs were arranged in a *U* shape around an easel of the sort favored by corporate presenters. The walls were plastered with the inspirational posters that I associated with twelve-step organizations. Several had photographs of Oprah Winfrey, perhaps the world's most famous yo-yo dieter, who invested $43 million in WW International in 2015.

> "Your Mind is Like a Parachute. It Only Works When It's Open."
>
> "I'm Not Here to Be Average. I'm Here to Be Awesome."
>
> "You Need Meetings. Meetings Need You."
>
> "Believe in Yourself!"

Eventually, two dozen of us settled into the chairs. It was obvious that everyone there knew each other, me being the exception. All the other attendees were female—not unusual for a WW session. We appeared to fall somewhere between forty and seventy years old, with most of us on the late-middle-aged end of that spectrum. We ranged from moderately heavy to morbidly obese.

Roseanne bustled in. Bustling, I soon learned, was her normal mode of locomotion. She looked to be in her fifties, and she'd permed her salt-and-pepper hair into close-cropped curls. Like all WW leaders, Roseanne had successfully lost weight on the program. Despite the absence of twenty-two pounds, she was by no means so slender as to present an impossible role model for us chubbies. Nor was she fat. Reassuringly solid came to mind. In the manner of most motivational speakers trained in the oratorical traditions of Dale Carnegie and Toastmasters International, Roseanne's delivery was painfully articulate, irrepressibly bubbly, and choreographed by exaggerated hand gestures and eye movements.

She launched right into a pep talk about mindsets. There were two, Roseanne told us: fixed and growth. Fixed would get us into trouble, especially when it came to losing weight. Such a mindset caused us to arbitrarily classify events as either good or bad, positive or negative. With fixed minds, we would quit WW if our attempts at controlling our appetites failed to show immediate results.

"You have the attitude that if you didn't lose weight last month, then you will never lose," she said. "You become discouraged." But, she added emphatically, we all had the ability shift our mindsets. She reminded us that the great Jean Nidetch, WW's founder, once said, "Nothing worthwhile is ever easy, but it can be a wonderful experience." The very fact that we were all in the room that morning was itself a sign that we were on the path toward the growth mindset. If you attain that mindset, when things go bad, you learn rather than get discouraged. Having the support of others was also helpful. "If there is no one else in your camp," she said, "we are in your camp."

At each subsequent weekly meeting, Roseanne lectured on a different subject. She told us that WW was permanent. Not a diet, but a lifestyle change. "We are in this for life," she said. "Who here thinks they will get to a point where they don't have to watch what they eat? We are all overweight."

One session was dedicated to defeating emotional eating. When we are happy, we eat to celebrate. When sad, to console ourselves. And when bored, to get excited. Food follows each emotion. We needed a plan for what we would do when hit by the pangs of emotional eating: call a friend, clean the junk drawer, read a magazine, play with a pet, watch television, dance to a favorite song. "The height of emotions does not last for long," she said. "Remember, you will get over it."

She told us to keep our "why close by." And that our whys should go beyond the numbers on those scales on the other side of the wall. The desire to lose twenty pounds was not enough. The more specific the reasons, the better. They could be athletic goals—running five kilometers. Or wanting to fit into a certain outfit. Or desiring to get off medications. To me, it all sounded like the stuff of AA meetings, only our desire for food, not booze, was the villain.

At the end of the session, Roseanne produced a slip of paper and held it aloft, as if preparing to read a proclamation. "As a group, we lost thirty-four pounds this week," she said, clapping her hands. We all joined her in giving ourselves a hearty round of applause. She presented one woman with a star-shaped Bravo sticker to place in her Success Story booklet, a reward for losing five pounds. Even louder applause resounded.

By attending those WW meetings, I was taking part in rituals that date back to 1961, when Jean Nidetch, a "Formerly Fat Housewife," as she called herself in her memoir, *The Story of Weight Watchers*, invited six "fat friends," over to her suburban Long Island apartment to talk about their mutual struggles to lose weight. At a younger stage in her life, Nidetch's peers would have probably voted her most likely to lead a life of quiet, working-class desperation. Instead, she became one of the most successful self-made American businesswomen of the twentieth century.

Nidetch grew up in a three-room Brooklyn apartment with her younger sister, mother, and father, who died when she was a first-year student at City College of New York. At age eighteen, she had to abandon the dream of a degree to help support her mother and sister by taking on a series of jobs, first at a furniture company, then at the publisher of a horse-racing tip sheet (the joint turned out to be clandestine, and the police closed it while she worked there), and finally at the Internal Revenue Service. She married three years after her father's death, and she and her husband eventually moved to Little Neck, on Long Island, where she settled into the life of a 1950s housewife, while he drove limousine buses and airport shuttles for a living.

In one way, Nidetch stood out: she was fat. She was born a medium-size, seven-pound three-ounce baby. "I started gaining weight the very next day," she wrote. And for decades she never stopped. As an adult, she was "married to fat man. Had a fat dog and fat friends. My whole world was fat." She and her husband, Marty (five foot ten and 265 pounds), were known as a jolly couple, the life of every party, always delighted to eat whatever a hostess served, and taking solace that at gatherings of their obese social circle, there was sure to be at least one even fatter couple.

She became what she described as a "professional dieter," repeatedly dropping twenty or thirty pounds and then packing them back on.

> I dieted in preparation for birthday parties. I dieted for graduation. I dieted for my engagement party. I dieted for my wedding. I'm talking about crash diets, any fast method, like black coffee with nothing. Or black coffee and cigarettes, or eggs and grapefruit. Oil capsules. Wafers that looked and tasted like dog biscuits. I took little red pills, little yellow pills, little green pills. I lost weight hundreds of times. You can lose weight if you eat watermelon for two weeks. Or bananas and milk, or cottage cheese and peaches. A neighbor tells you about a diet and it works. You lose weight. Sometimes you don't feel well, often you don't look well, but you always lose weight.
>
> I remember one diet where I drank oil and evaporated milk, cold, three times a day, and you mixed it in a plastic container.... I definitely lost weight. I also got sick to my stomach constantly. My skin had a funny color and my nails got soft.

At age thirty-eight, Nidetch stood five foot seven, weighed 214 pounds (she never publicly admitted to more than 145), and wore size forty-four dresses. She hit bottom (or, more accurately, hit the top) while pushing her shopping cart down the aisle of a supermarket and encountered an acquaintance whom she despised. "You look marvelous," the woman said, hardly bothering to mask her insincerity. "When are you due?"

Nidetch was not pregnant.

That same afternoon, she made an appointment to visit the New York City Department of Health Obesity Clinic, overseen by Dr. Norman Jolliffe, who was known internationally for his work in public health and as the author of the book *Reduce and Stay Reduced.* Jolliffe called his weight-loss program the Prudent Diet. He based it on the erroneous theory that the human body possessed an "appestat," which turned off hunger when someone had eaten adequately, much like a thermostat turns off a furnace when a room reaches a set temperature. The appestats of fat people, he contended, were broken and failed to switch over to the off position after the consumption of sufficient food.

His clinic enforced a rigid approach to peeling pounds off the doctor's patients. A slender woman greeted Nidetch, glanced at her figure, and brusquely decreed that she would weigh 142 pounds—not an ounce more or less—if she adhered to the organization's program. To do so, she had to eat exactly the foods prescribed. The slightest deviation was forbidden, and the penalty for even a minor infraction (and not losing weight at the expected rate was considered ipso facto evidence that you were cheating) was getting kicked out of the program, to be replaced by a more dedicated participant drawn from the clinic's lengthy waiting list.

Nidetch dropped twenty pounds in ten weeks, but that displeased the slender group leader, who told her that she should have done better. Nidetch was busted. She'd religiously adhered to the diet in all areas but one: cookies. She could not live without them. She secreted cookies in the glove compartment of her car for nibbling while behind the wheel and kept a stash of cookies in her bathroom, where she could cheat in privacy. As disciplined as she was about all of Jolliffe's other dietary edicts, she could not kick her cookie addiction.

In addition to being fat throughout her life, Nidetch had always been an accomplished blabbermouth. Frustrated by her inability to resist cookies, she decided to confess her weakness to six of her fat friends. Gathering in her apartment, they discovered that they battled many similar demons. Food fixations and cravings were normal for these overweight people. One woman shared that she kept her tins of nuts in the pantry behind the canned asparagus, knowing that her kids would never venture there. Another hid éclairs in the oven. A third stashed her candy behind the beef in the freezer. Most admitted to waking in the middle of the night, tiptoeing downstairs, and sneaking a little something from the fridge or freezer.

Although Nidetch had promised not to alter the clinic's diet in any way, she did add one ingredient: talk. By talking together, she and her friends discovered they had more power over themselves. Chatting with the group helped Nidetch overcome her need to dash to the bathroom every time she felt the urge to eat a cookie. It helped her stay on the clinic's diet.

Nidetch was ahead of her time. Only recently have researchers come to understand the advantages of joining a group versus solo therapy in what psychologists call behavioral acknowledgment programs. And for Nidetch, the weight fell away. Within a year, she had lost 72 pounds, plateauing at 142 (that snippy clinic woman had been right) and staying within a few pounds of that number for the rest of her life. Her husband lost 70 pounds.

Other members of her little impromptu group also found themselves losing weight and keeping it off for the first time in their lives. They began meeting at her place every week, with extra gatherings on Saturday mornings to gird themselves against the temptations of weekend parties. They told their obese friends about the miracles that were occurring at Nidetch's apartment, and the group grew, moving first into the cellar of her building and then to an abandoned synagogue. She started to charge participants a nominal amount to cover her expenses, but her get-togethers remained a hobby until April 1963 when she registered Weight Watchers as a business and begin charging an admission fee of two dollars per session.

Driven by Nidetch's natural talents as a saleswoman and public speaker, her "little club" boomed. Within a decade a total of more than twenty thousand classes were being held each month in forty-nine states, as well as Canada, Germany, and South Africa. When the company went public, Nidetch became an instant multimillionaire. Weight Watchers had more than four hundred employees and sold magazines, cookbooks, frozen foods, and even a line of official scales upon which members could weigh themselves. Nidetch became a celebrity, speaking before sold-out theater audiences and appearing on morning television and late-night talk shows.

In the early days, while offering the support of regular talk sessions, Nidetch adhered strictly to the draconian regime endured by patients at Dr. Jolliffe's clinic. Members had to obey set rules. They could not skip any meals; nor could they make substitutions to the prescribed menu. She forbade them from counting calories. "We may eat all we like, but not the foods we ate before," Nidetch wrote. "Not the foods that made us fat."

Foods were either "mandatory," "allowed," "or "prohibited." The long list of banned food and drink included bananas, cherries, avocados, corn, mayonnaise, potatoes, rice, spaghetti, sugar, and alcohol. Nidetch demanded that participants eat liver at least once a week (permitting members to choose between beef, lamb, or chicken liver). Women had to eat one slice (men, two slices) of enriched white or whole-wheat bread at breakfast and lunch, but never dinner. Everyone had to consume at least four eggs a week, but no more than seven, and their diet also had to include either beef, hot dogs, lamb, turkey (dark meat only, with skin removed), or salmon three times a week.

Nidetch imposed restrictions on who could join. No one who was less that ten pounds overweight was allowed through the doors. This

NIDETCH

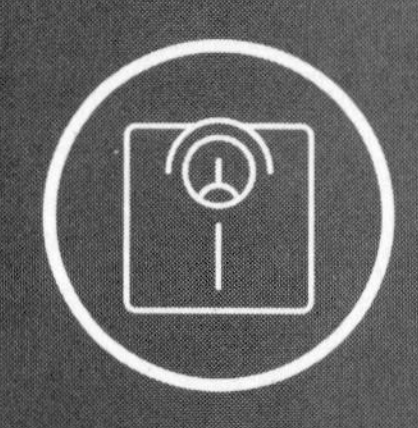

JEAN NIDETCH

FOUNDER OF WEIGHT WATCHERS
(NOW WW INTERNATIONAL)

OBJECTIVE

INITIAL AND SUSTAINED
WEIGHT LOSS

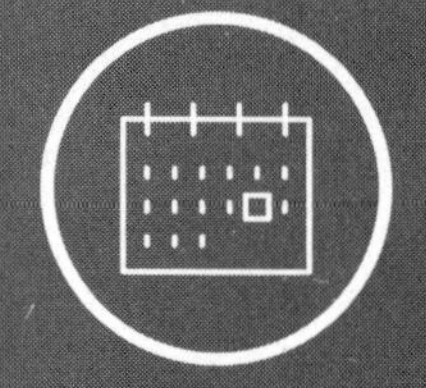

APPROACH

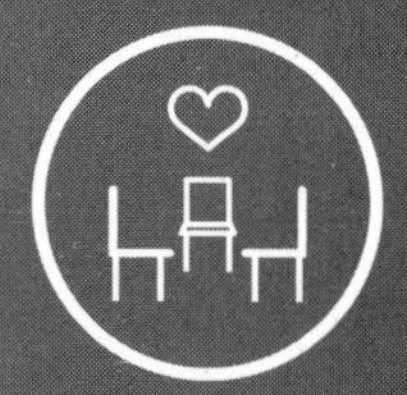

STRICT ADHERENCE
TO PROGRAM

REINFORCEMENT &
SUPPORT THROUGH
COMMUNITY

deterred curiosity seekers and so prevented heavier members from becoming intimidated or feeling ashamed. Upon admittance, she told new members exactly what their eventual goal weight would be, just as the woman at the clinic had given Nidetch a goal. She encouraged Weight Watchers to keep a "fat picture" of themselves with them at all times, and to paste another on the refrigerator door to remind them of the bad old days, in case they were tempted to indulge in a scoop of ice cream or slice of leftover cake.

Many of Nidetch's original rules seem passé and occasionally humorous, but other precepts of her original diet plan remain in force. My group's leader, Roseanne, like all others before her, had successfully lost weight on the program and kept the pounds off. (In the early days, leaders were fired if they gained more than two pounds.) Like original Weight Watchers, we were told that we had embarked upon a "new way to live." We would gain "power over ourselves." We were engaged in a "war" with obesity, and we would have to eat the WW way for the rest of our lives.

Although I wasn't asked to keep a "fat picture" on hand, we all weighed in before each meeting. But even that ritual has since become optional. Nidetch believed that the scale, as cruel and callous as its dial could be, was the only way to measure a diet's success. Mercifully, the employees who sat at the desk beside the intimidating WW scale that I stepped on prior to each session refrained from broadcasting the readings to the group at large, an earlier policy. Convinced that her members responded to material rewards, Nidetch began giving out custom-made pins of real gold to women and gold tie clips to men who lost ten pounds, with additional genuine diamond chips inserted for every subsequent ten-pound loss. "I can't tell you why I gave the awards," Nidetch wrote. "Except that when your child has done something you're proud of, you've got to reward him." These days, successful WW members receive reward stickers and shiny charms made out of a silvery metal—definitely not of the precious kind. We also earned Wellness Wins points for attending meetings, losing weight, exercising, and keeping careful track of our food consumption. We could accumulate points and trade them in for free membership, as well as for water bottles, clothing, and other WW merch.

This kinder, gentler WW reflects another trait embedded in the company's DNA and no doubt contributes to its longevity—a chameleonlike ability to adapt to the latest trend and to copy the successes of competitors such as Jenny Craig and Nutrisystem and, eventually, South Beach, The Whole30, mobile apps, and Fitbit. The adaptability allowed WW to weather a series of financial swings that saw its earnings soar and then plummet, only to rise again. The price of the company's stock took the same trajectory.

In the late 1970s, the firm, having been sold to what was then the H. J. Heinz Company (now the Kraft Heinz Company) for $72 million, rolled out a PepStep program, which introduced walking and other gentle exercise to the original diet. Shortly thereafter, Weight Watchers began allowing participants to make substitutions to its rigid menu. To make it simpler for customers to monitor their food intake, each member received a set number of points per day, based on a formula that included calories, carbohydrates, fat, and fiber. By 2018, the mere mention of the word *diet* had become politically incorrect as the world entered what Weight Watchers called the postdiet age. It was then that Weight Watchers changed its name to WW International, insisting that the company was suddenly no longer about losing weight, and instead about "Wellness that Works." With the new slogan, WW would expand beyond the scale to build healthy habits without focusing on weight loss. It did, however, hedge its bets by appending the tagline "Weight Watchers Reimagined" to its new WW International logo. Along with the name change came alterations in other established Weight Watchers terminology. The "meetings" I was attending every week became "workshops." I no longer had to submit to a "weigh-in" before each workshop but could stand on the scales for an optional "wellness check-in." The "store" in which we assembled was now called a "studio." And Roseanne, our effervescent "leader," had a new title, "wellness coach."

For me, and I suspect many others, the reason I was paying WW more than fifty dollars a month was to lose weight. Wellness sounded nice and all, but as far as I was concerned, I was still a Weight Watcher, and getting skinnier reigned paramount. To accomplish that, I still had to stay within a daily quota of SmartPoints, based on my age, gender, and weight. Keeping at or below that limit would allow me to reach an interim goal arbitrarily set by WW, a manageable loss of about fifteen pounds. I wanted to lose more, but setting a too ambitious goal might make me discouraged with my progress and more likely to drop out.

Every food item was worth a fixed number of these points. I was to "track," in WW parlance, everything I swallowed, with the goal of never exceeding my daily quota (although the program permitted a small weekly surplus to compensate for the occasional slip). In the pre-cell-phone era, this might have been a daunting chore, but my tuition included access to an app that allowed me to look up the point value of any food I could imagine, including all manner of packaged items from the supermarket and menu offerings from popular restaurant chains. I merely had to enter the food, and the app kept track of my daily total. Little wonder that WW has been a repeat winner for *U.S. News & World Report*'s annual "Easiest Diet to Follow" rankings.

But what was the science behind these user-friendly "points"?

Who better to answer that question than Gary Foster, WW's chief scientific officer? Foster works from the company's Midtown Manhattan headquarters, a spare, utilitarian workspace for the executives of a billion-dollar-plus corporation. I found that reassuring. My monthly payments were not being squandered on pampering the denizens at the top. Foster, who wore a navy blue blazer over an open shirt, was balding, tall, and had the slim physique of someone fortunate enough (or well-disciplined enough) to never have a need for the services offered by his employer. Foster spoke in the measured cadence of a professor—a good professor who was aware of the importance of his subject and eager that students understand. Indeed, he'd been an academic for more than two decades and was the founder and head of the Center for Obesity Research and Education at Temple University, in Philadelphia, before assuming his WW post. Call me naïve, but I had expected that the chief scientific officer of a company dedicated, in a large part, to weight loss would have a background in gastroenterology, metabolism biology, or at least be a registered dietitian. But Foster's PhD is in psychology—which says a lot about the scientific underpinnings of what was happening during those sessions I sat through, listening to Roseanne. "My union card is in psychology," he told me. "But I caught the obesity bug in my mid-twenties. What captivated my curiosity and passion was helping people struggling with their weight. Weight management is about biology, metabolic rates, and so on, but a lot of it is about behavior training."

The younger Foster was all about research. He did the first controlled, randomized scientific study on the Atkins Diet. (He confirmed to me that participants lost weight faster than a control group in the early months, but were no better off after a year.) Eventually, he became interested in finding practical applications to weight-loss research, what he called "scalable solutions." He started working with the National Institutes of Health, insurance companies, and school systems on ways to reduce obesity, but remained unsatisfied. "I was published three or four times in the *Journal of the American Medical Association*. I was on the *Today* show. The papers I wrote had great press exposure. And all of that had no impact. Zero. Zilch," he told me.

By taking the job at WW, he found a real-world outlet for his scholarly research. "You won't find many companies that are as well grounded in science as WW," he said. "We don't consider financials and spreadsheets until we can say, 'what we are about to do is a credible scientific proposition.' It sounds corny, but we leverage science. There's not a single bit of understatement there from my point of view. We develop a program, and immediately 3.5 million people will be on that program. And we'll get an immediate read on the results. It's an opportunity to have a big impact."

Foster and I met just as he was rolling out WW's Freestyle plan, which has since been replaced with a program called MyWW. He explained that the diet was still based on the tried-and-true SmartPoints, which simplify complex nutritional information on those government-mandated food labels I never bother to read, and, the FDA admits, most consumers do not understand. Points are still built on a foundation of the number of calories each item contains, but with some key refinements. Sugar and fat content increase the number of points, regardless of the number of calories. Protein lowers points. A Hershey's milk chocolate candy bar has 214 calories and is worth 6 WW points, while a four-ounce steak having roughly the same number of calories, but with less sugar and more protein, "costs" only 4 points. Similarly, you get only 1 point if your breakfast is a Greek yogurt and fruit parfait but 12 (about half of most members' daily allotment) if you opt for two pancakes with chocolate chips and maple syrup, even though both breakfasts have the same number of calories. To make the program easier to follow, many foods have zero points. In theory, you can eat all you want of vegetables, fruits, skinless chicken breast, skinless turkey breast, nonfat yogurt, eggs, seafood, beans, peas, lentils, tofu, and corn—all zero-point fare.

WW INTERNATIONAL POINTS SYSTEM AT-A-GLANCE

COUNTING POINTS INSTEAD OF CALORIES FOR WEIGHT CONTROL AND HEALTH BENEFITS.

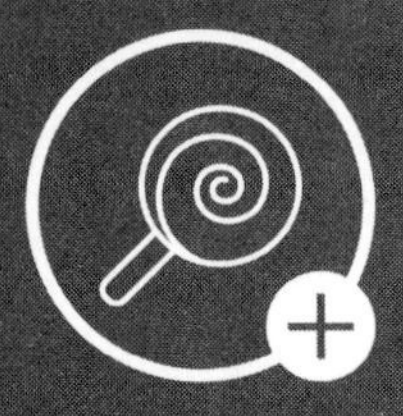

FOODS WITH SUGAR AND FAT CONTENTS EQUAL HIGH POINTS.

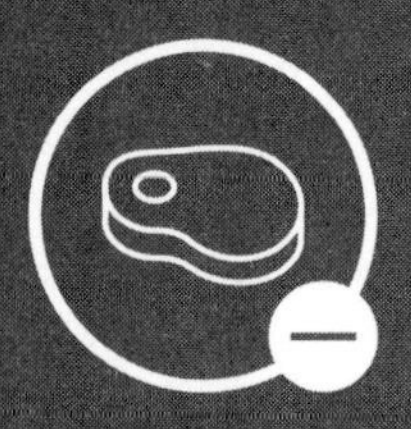

FOODS WITH HIGHER PROTEIN CONTENT HAVE LOWER POINTS.

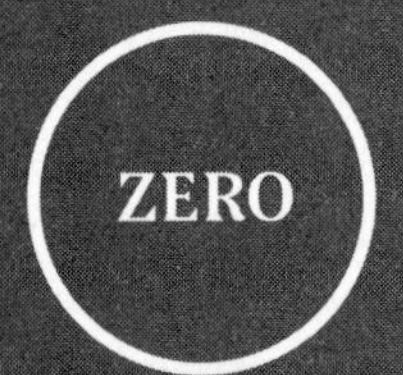

MANY LOW-FAT, NO-SUGAR, HIGH-PROTEIN FOODS EQUAL ZERO POINTS.

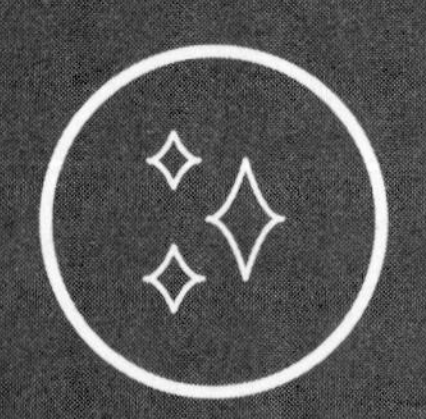

"WEEKLIES": BONUS POINT ALLOWANCES FOR THE OCCASIONAL SPLURGE WHILE OTHERWISE STAYING WITHIN THE RECOMMENDED TOTAL POINTS.

"Does that mean I can eat five eggs for breakfast and still be compliant?" I asked Foster.

"Yes," he said, with a knowing smile. "But our research shows that if people really do things like that, they don't do so often or for long. If they continued, that would be a problem, but it tends to take care of itself. Essentially, we're telling people that zero-point items are something you don't have to expend a lot of mental gymnastics on. We're worried about the higher-point-valued foods."

Points aside, calories are still important in the WW program, even if they are not emphasized. "You have to eat fewer calories than you burn to lose weight," Foster said, invoking the traditional thinking of nutritionist experts. "We're not defying the laws of thermodynamics here. What we're saying is that calories are only part of the picture. Purely for weight loss, you can eat a thousand calories of candy or a thousand calories of broccoli—though neither would be nutritionally recommended—and you'll still lose weight. But you wouldn't get the important health benefit consumers want. That's why points take into consideration more than calories."

Talking with Foster made it clear that when losing pounds the WW way, what went on inside my brain was as important as what went into my belly. "Half the battle of trying to manage weight has nothing to do with eating. It's mindset," said Foster. *Mindset* was only one of many bits of psychological jargon Forster dropped into his explanation of the WW program. He also spoke of "behavior acknowledgment," "cognitive cushions," "stimulus control," "external triggers," "empirically tested behavioral phenomena," and "bringing positive psychology to the masses."

Much of the system is designed to act as subtle, even subconscious, persuasion. Foster said the organization no longer resorted to words like *have to*, *must*, or *should* in guiding customers to a better way of eating. "Those words sound very diet-y," he said. "They make it feel like a death sentence, rather than a way to live the rest of your life. Our methods make you feel better. It's that simple."

So instead of issuing direct commands and ultimatums, WW uses SmartPoints to encourage members to favor certain categories of foods, such as fruits, vegetables, and lean meats that help reduce weight and bring additional health benefits. Going out to a restaurant and devouring a slab of prime rib is perfectly fine, according to Foster, but WW members have to balance the pleasure such indulgences deliver against their cost in points (about fifteen for prime rib). If it's worth it, go ahead. Otherwise, consider ordering the grilled salmon instead.

The new points allotment also includes what the company calls weeklies, or bonus points, which you can draw on and still remain compliant should you overdo it one day. Foster compares these weeklies to a bank account that you can dip into if need be. WW added weeklies because one of the main reasons participants abandon the program is that they become discouraged and give up when they fall off the wagon. The bank account allows people to stay engaged. And fear not, Foster's crew has done the math so people like me can sin a little bit, but still lose weight.

Peer-reviewed research lends credence to the company's claims that WW works for many participants. Foster made sure I left our meeting with a sheaf of a dozen photocopied journal articles. It came as no surprise that each of them, in one way or another, attested to the WW program's scientific grounding. Papers in such respected academic publications as the *Journal of the American Medical Association*, *Lancet*, *BMJ* (formerly *British Medical Journal*), *Annals of Internal Medicine*, and the *Journal of American Medicine* confirmed that my $54.95 monthly WW dues was not a complete waste of money. Compared to those who tried to diet on their own or with medical supervision, WW members dropped more weight (about ten pounds after a year, on average) and kept it off for at least a year. The *American Journal of Medicine* concluded that WW members were eight times more likely to lose between 5 and 10 percent of their body weight than those opting for self-help.

At WW, scientific research is also weighed against the company's formidable body of consumer research. "We are a science-based company," Foster said. "But we try to understand the cultural zeitgeist. What's the consumer sentiment around losing weight? If we are not in sync with the zeitgeist, we could have the most efficacious program in the world, and nobody would be willing to engage with it." Getting members engaged and keeping them that way is critical to WW's survival. Before messing with success by rolling out the Freestyle changes, the company commissioned a six-month clinical trial conducted by Deborah Tate, of the University of North Carolina's Weight Research Program. She found that participants not only lost an average of nearly 8 percent of their body weight but also had lower blood pressure and improved stamina and flexibility, even while they reported a decrease in food cravings. Virtually all of the participants claimed to be satisfied with the new program, saying that it helped them feel better and was simple to follow.

Roseanne was good at her job. I left that first workshop equipped with my new WW app, inspired to start shedding pounds. To my surprise, I found electronically tracking every morsel I ate interesting in a nerdish way—at first. A few taps of the WW app on my phone brought up the point value of each food item. The device took care of the rote mathematical legwork of keeping my daily tally and even had a handy chart that told me at a glance how close I was to hitting my limit.

However, from the outset I encountered one annoying (and perverse, given WW's commitment to healthful eating) difficulty. While the app provided instant information for every packaged processed food and every item on the menus of chain restaurants, figuring out points for from-scratch recipes involved entering each individual ingredient and providing precise quantities. Look up Olive Garden's chicken Alfredo, and you instantly find that it's worth 27 points. (Yikes, there goes the daily limit.) Figuring out the point value of my own homemade version involved finding and adding together the points in ¼ cup of butter (4), 1 cup of heavy cream (16), and 1½ cups of grated Parmesan cheese (12). Thank God the garlic and parsley I used in the dish are zero pointers and didn't have to be considered. I added up those numbers, for a total of 32, then divided it by four servings to arrive at 8 points. After all that tapping, I'd kind of lost my appetite for Alfredo.

Nonetheless, I dutifully soldiered along, keeping careful track of everything. I even went so far as digging out an old shot glass from the back of a cabinet to carefully mete out a pre-dinner cocktail of 1½ ounces of bourbon (2 points), versus my former custom of pouring liberally until the liquor rose to the top of three or four ice cubes, which would have been worth who knows how many points. For one solid week, I kept to my allotted points.

When I reported back to the WW studio, the scale showed that I'd dropped six pounds in my first seven days as a Weight Watcher. Roseanne singled me out, clapping her hands and telling the room that I, the newbie, had lost six pounds. She peeled one of the star-shaped Bravo stickers off her roll and handed it to me to affix to the proper spot in my Success Story booklet.

Tracking my food intake with the WW app soon lost its novelty. What had initially been kind of cool became a duty, then a chore. I took shortcuts, failing to type in every ingredient in every dish I prepared. The shot glass languished in the liquor cabinet. I began filling my wine glasses to their former level, figuring an ounce or two in excess of the five that WW considered to be a serving wouldn't hurt. Sometimes a day would go by when I neglected to tally my points, and I was left to track my meals from memory, which, as any expert will tell you, is notoriously unreliable when it comes to matters of food and drink, even with the best intentions.

That WW scale, a stern taskmaster if ever there was one, punished me on my third visit. I'd regained two of the six pounds lost the previous week. There was no applause for me at the end of that meeting. I tried to be much more diligent the following week, but was disappointed to see that my efforts resulted in eliminating only one of those two regained pounds. I put on another pound during week four. Roseanne gave me a little one-month metal charm to affix to a bracelet, if I was a charm-bracelet kind of guy. I felt undeserving. By then, I was down only two pounds, at a cost of about twenty-five bucks each, given the monthly membership fee. At that rate, I would have to part with $1,000 to reach a level that would make Doctor Dennis smile.

I stuck with the program for another month, but I found it inconvenient to get to meetings. Tracking went by the wayside. I finally went to WW's website and cancelled the automatic renewal to the program, something that was refreshingly straightforward, to the company's credit. My email inbox continues to fill with special offers enjoining me to return.

Despite my own failure to become permanently thinner as a Weight Watcher, all that tracking instilled one valuable lesson: I call it Barry's Big Sin Theory of Weight Management, although I suspect that Roseanne and Gary Foster would shriek at the name. Day after day, my cell phone showed me that I could usually stay within my SmartPoint limit—not mindlessly, but with modest effort by relying on a little old-fashioned willpower—so long as I did not touch a drop of alcohol or a piece of cheese, two items I loved dearly. Consuming one or the other—or often a smidgeon of both—inevitably put me a few points over the line. On days when I poured generously, without measuring, or simply took a wild guess at how much my slice of Camembert weighed (when was the last time you weighted a sliver of cheese?), I'm sure my overage was greater than I estimated.

Hearing about the challenges and listening to stories of relapses shared by cronies during what I came to think of as the show-and-tell session during each meeting, indicated that my WW classmates all committed their own Big Sins, just like Nidetch's original group, though my transgressions were the only ones that involved excess corn liquor. For one woman, it was excellent, gooey pizza from the restaurant she drove past every day just before dinner on her way home from work. In her exhausted state, picking up a couple of pizza pies was a lot faster and convenient (albeit more caloric) than cooking for her family. Another had a weakness for Ben and Jerry's cookie dough ice cream. One couldn't get behind the wheel of her car without a can of regular Coke and a bag of salt and vinegar potato chips. One watched a great deal of television after dinner, munching the whole time. Sinners all, we Weight Watchers.

Maybe it was time I gave up on dieting. A couple of years had passed since my appointment with Doctor Dennis. I'd tried more than a dozen weight-loss programs, given them all a fair shake, and ended up right back where I started, still carting around the same damn forty unwanted pounds. Why couldn't I just eat? Plenty of other cultures do.

CHAPTER EIGHT

HILL TRIBE

In Spanish, *Loma Linda* means "beautiful hill." I guess the name and the town's reputation as an American Shangri-La, where a strikingly large percentage of residents enjoy exceptionally long, vigorous lives had led me to believe that I would be visiting an earthly paradise. Those visions were put sorely to the test as I drove toward the town of about twenty-five thousand an hour east of Los Angeles. I couldn't imagine a more frustrating way to experience the Sixth Circle of California Freeway Hell. All manner of tractor-trailer trucks, flatbeds, oil tankers, and concrete mixers barreled along at heart-stopping speeds, pinning my tinny rental car between them, belching gray clouds of diesel exhaust, and creating a cacophony of roaring air brakes, gunning engines, and whining tires. Braver, or more foolish, drivers than I cut in and out of the few precious inches of life-saving margin that I tried to maintain between my fragile conveyance and the behemoths on all sides of me.

Until we all stopped. And stayed stopped. Minutes crept by. I drummed my fingers and inhaled fumes, becalmed amid the waves of heat rising from a twelve-lane isthmus of asphalt dividing an ocean of warehouses, box stores, railyards, and fast-food joints. Gazing ahead, I could barely make out the jagged profile of the San Bernardino Mountains, all but obscured by dull, brownish haze. It struck me that Loma Linda's residents must have achieved their longevity despite, not because of, their pretty hill's location in Los Angeles's smoggy backyard. There must have been some pretty powerful forces for good health at work.

I'd made an appointment to talk to Dr. Gary Fraser, a professor of epidemiology at Loma Linda University School of Public Health. His office is in a large, rambling building with beige stucco sides and a red tile roof. The university's campus is, indeed, set atop a beautiful hill, with curving streets bordered by gardens and shaded by palm trees, all bathed in golden sunlight unfiltered by the smog, which miraculously seemed to lift when I pulled onto the exit ramp from the freeway.

In 2011, *Newsweek* published an infographic with the tongue-in-cheek headline "How to Live Forever." One option, according to the magazine, was to reside in Loma Linda. As I listened to Fraser describe the healthy habits and longevity of the townspeople, I began to think maybe it wasn't quite so tongue-in-cheek. "Something real is going on here," he told me.

That is an understatement. Author Dan Buettner identified Loma Linda as the only locale in the United States that he considers one of the world's Blue Zones, his term for the handful of places where living one hundred years and beyond is common. For his 2008 book, *The Blue Zones: 9 Lessons for Living Longer from the People Who Live the Longest,* Buettner made a quick trip to Loma Linda. While there, he rode shotgun with Marge Jetton, 103 years old at the time, as she lead-footed her Caddy through the bumper-to-bumper traffic on I-10, racing from one volunteer commitment to the next in her packed schedule—this was after an hour of pedaling a stationary bike and lifting dumbbells. He watched 94-year-old Dr. Ellsworth Wareham wiping sweat from his brow while digging postholes for a new fence around his yard. The next morning, Wareham, a surgeon, went off to his job performing open-heart surgery with a team at the hospital. Despite his advanced years, younger colleagues insisted he be there. They valued his steady hands and the storehouse of knowledge that enabled him to perform any part of the intricate operations. Buettner also spent time with Minnie Wood (100), Letha Graham (102), and a feisty, though somewhat hard-of-hearing, Ethyl Meilicke (108). All of these seniors lived within a few miles of each other.

When Professor Rhonda Spencer-Hwang of Loma Linda University wanted to conduct a study that necessitated finding a cohort of extremely old people and lacked funding for travel, it posed no problem. She easily recruited ten centenarians from her immediate circle of acquaintances in the community, along with several other subjects in their late nineties with all indications that they, too, would achieve 100. None of them looked a day over 80. They lived independently. They suffered from no chronic diseases. Spencer-Hwang's oldest subject was one of her husband's aunts, who was still active at 105, although her family had confiscated her car keys when she was 101, not because her driving skills had diminished but because she took a fall while stepping over the threshold to her garage.

It is no coincidence that nearly a third of the residents of Loma Linda are practicing Seventh-day Adventists, a Christian denomination started in 1863 in Battle Creek, Michigan, by a group that included Ellen G. White (see page 39), thought by followers to be a prophet who received messages directly from God. White's writings have had lasting effects on Adventist doctrine. She believed that the body and soul were one and that corporal health was directly linked to spiritual health. "You are the temple of the Holy Spirit," according to 1 Corinthians. Believers, therefore, have a moral responsibility to treat their bodies with reverence and take good care of them by getting plenty of exercise, shunning tobacco, and avoiding alcohol, meat, caffeine, and spices.

For more than 150 years, Seventh-day Adventists have lived according to their church's edicts on diet and health. For them, White's words need no scientific validation. But their benefits have been confirmed by the largest and most detailed epidemiological studies undertaken anywhere. With origins that date back seven decades, the ongoing Adventist Health Study, which Fraser oversees, has followed nearly 150,000 members of the church in the United States and Canada.

The results leave little doubt that White was onto something profound. In California, Adventist men thirty years of age live about 7.3 years longer than the average Caucasian California male (85.3 years versus 78). Women live 4.4 years longer. Among the many Adventists who are strict vegetarians, the gap is larger, 9.5 years for men and 6.1 years for women. For Adventists of any age, the chances of dying are about 35 percent lower than for the rest of us. More than 300 peer-reviewed scientific articles based on the Adventist studies have been published in respected medical journals such as *The New England Journal of Medicine*, *American Journal of Epidemiology*, and *American Journal of Clinical Nutrition*.

The origins of the Adventist study go back to 1951, when Dr. Mervyn Hardinge began conducting research into the nutritional effects of the vegetarian diet practiced by his fellow Adventists. His early work met resistance from some church leaders, who asked whether Adventists really wanted to submit beliefs delivered from God to a statistical evaluation. They feared that if Hardinge's results showed deficiencies in the diet espoused by White and early Adventists, it would embarrass the church. But eventually they agreed, feeling that if White's doctrines were worth adhering to, they were worth subjecting to rigorous scientific scrutiny. They needn't have worried. After proving to a then-skeptical academic community that vegetarians could get all the nutrition they required, Hardinge went on to found the Loma Linda University School of Public Health. (He died in 2010, at age ninety-six.)

In 1987, Hardinge recruited Fraser to take over the Adventist study. Originally trained as a cardiologist, Fraser, like Dean Ornish, became discouraged after being unable to help patients who came to him suffering from the consequences of a lifetime of smoking and poor diet. He switched to epidemiology, hoping to do research that could prevent the conditions he had encountered while practicing his original specialty.

I hoped Fraser would answer two main questions: One, would he provide me with detailed background on the study's findings; and two, was there anything from the results that those of us who are not followers of the Adventist religious beliefs could adopt.

Fraser was a good advertisement for the Adventist lifestyle. He was seventy-two years old when we met, but I would have guessed that he was at least a decade younger, with his trim physique and crisply parted salt-and-pepper hair. He told me he planned to stay in his leadership position until he turned seventy-five and then he'd see how it was going. "Maybe I'll go part-time. There doesn't seem to be a lot of sense in retiring," he said, his twangy vowels betraying a New Zealand upbringing, despite the passage of fifty years since he first came to the United States.

He outlined some of his study's findings:

- → Only about half of the modern-day Adventists in the study were vegetarians, some of whom adhered to lacto-ovo practices, meaning their diet included eggs and dairy products.
- → Those Adventists who reported that they ate meat consumed it rarely.
- → Not being obese was more important to subjects' health than avoiding animal products.
- → Thinner subjects, vegetarian or not, outlived their more corpulent peers.
- → The more that subjects relied on plant products for their nourishment, the longer and healthier their lives. Fraser suspects that it has something to do with the phytochemicals in fruits and vegetables that protect against cancer.
- → Those in the study who ate red meat regularly had a greater chance of experiencing heart attacks, regardless of other factors in their favor. "Even if we adjust for the differences in weight, what people eat still has an impact," he said.
- → Adventists who refrained from snacking, dined less frequently and earlier in the day, and had breakfast as their largest meal, weighed less than their counterparts.
- → Longer-lived participants got regular exercise, but it did not have to be strenuous.
- → Virtually no Adventists smoked, and many abstained from alcohol.

But the most startling finding—and one that would have strained my credulity had it not been replicated in several independent studies and controlled experiments—is that regularly eating nuts of any kind (even

DO THIS

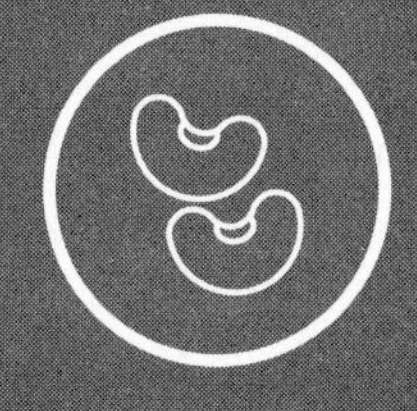

NUTS

VEGETARIAN OR
MINIMAL MEAT

UNPROCESSED
FOODS

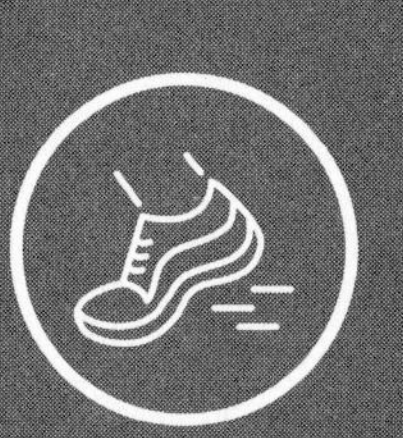

REGULAR
MODERATE EXERCISE

NOT THIS

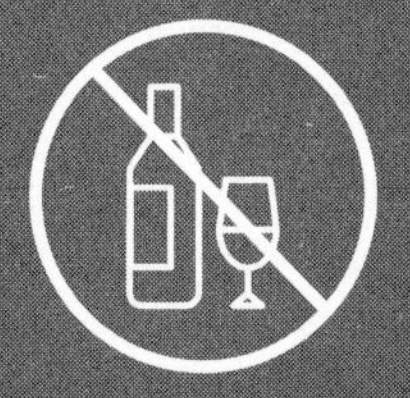

DRINKING
ALCOHOL

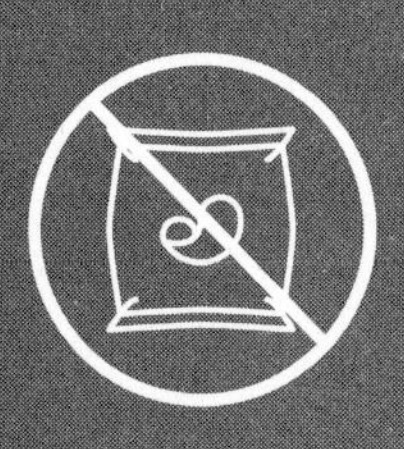

SNACKING

SMOKING

peanuts, which are actually legumes) can add years to your life by significantly reducing the risk of heart disease. When Fraser first observed this trend, it was greeted with skepticism by fellow scientists, who rightly pointed out that nuts were high in fats, which were believed to cause cardiac disease. But Fraser's evidence showed that heart disease was about 50 percent lower among those who ate nuts about five times a week. But not too many. "A dozen or so nuts a day is sufficient," Fraser told me. "Nuts do have a lot of calories, so if you sit in front of the television and eat an entire can, you're not going to be in very good shape." The explanation for why nuts are beneficial has yet to be confirmed, but Fraser said that studies show that in general, the unsaturated fats in nuts tend to lower cholesterol and improve blood chemistry. But he suspects that something other than the "good" fats in nuts must be at play. "The protein in nuts may also be heart-healthy," he said.

Fraser practices what he preaches. An Adventist since birth, he was raised as a lacto-ovo vegetarian, although he occasionally strayed and consumed red meat, particularly during his grueling years as an on-call medical resident in Auckland, putting in twenty-four-hour shifts and eating dinner late at night, when New Zealand's ubiquitous lamb was the only thing left in the hospital cafeteria. Today he will have the occasional piece of fish, but he eats no red meat. Chicken is also off his menu, not because his studies have linked it to poor health outcomes but because he is morally against the way chickens are raised in modern industrial farms. "I used to keep chickens as a kid. I think the industrial way of keeping them is a sin," he said. He does not drink alcohol and has never in his life inhaled a puff of tobacco smoke.

For breakfast on the day we met, he had eaten granola in soy milk, topped by grapes and unsalted roasted almonds—his favorite nuts. On other mornings, he might top his granola with berries. His lunch, he said, is "very boring." It consists of three slices of bread (always whole-wheat), spread with margarine or olive oil. One slice is topped with raw tomatoes; one with half a banana, mashed; and the third with chopped dates, to which he is very partial. Dinner is often a vegetarian stir-fry using a minimal amount of fat, with perhaps some chopped potatoes or a soy-based meat replacement. "Foods that are somewhat appetizing and not mass-produced," he said. "When you are brought up on a good vegetarian diet by someone who knows how to cook, you don't really miss meat."

I suppose I could change my diet to be more like Fraser's but, in other ways, I cannot emulate Adventists. They have a profound spiritual life, which I lack. The last time I attended a church service was more than two decades ago, when we had my youngest daughter confirmed as a Catholic, under intense lobbying from her devout grandmother. Adventists are adamant about observing the Sabbath; they do no work and reserve the day for church services and coming together with friends and family for meals. Sundays too often find me on deadline at my desk. My family is far flung, and our gatherings occur only a few times a year. For the Adventists, living among like-minded members of a congregation provides social and practical support for maintaining a vegetarian diet, as do the products available at local grocery stores and restaurants.

"So," I asked Fraser with some trepidation, "based on the studies, is there hope for us non-Adventists?"

"Oh, yeah," he said. "I am not an evangelist. Physiologically, we are not any different from you. High blood pressure, cholesterol, smoking, past smoking—we find all these things in our population. We are fairly ordinary Americans, and even with modest changes, non-Adventists can benefit."

Fraser feels that, ideally, everybody should eat a plant-based diet, but doesn't go so far as to insist that we all become vegans. "Our analyses show a mixed picture when we compare Adventist lacto-ovo vegetarians with our vegans," he said. "But what is clear is that both of these eating patterns have advantages over consuming meat."

In an independent examination of the Adventist Health Study, Harvard's Dr. Walter Willett concluded that "no history of smoking, avoidance of overweight, and a vegetarian diet" were keys to a long life, but "the magnitude of benefit for regular consumption of nuts, lean body mass, and regular exercise was greater than vegetarian status itself."

To find the other Blue Zones described in his book, Buettner had to travel to such far-flung corners of the planet as Okinawa, Japan; Italy's island of Sardinia; Costa Rica's Nicoya Peninsula; and the Greek island of Ikaria. His interviews with aged residents of each of these regions interested me in an abstract way, but I had trouble applying the secrets of long life from impoverished farmers in places like Sardinia to my own lifestyle in the United States, where I don't have to scramble over scrubby mountainsides in pursuit of sheep and goats to scratch out a living, or limit the amount of meat in my diet because there is simply none to be had. Loma Linda, on the other hand, was on the outskirts of the second biggest metropolitan area in the United States. People there looked like my friends, neighbors, and colleagues—just older. They lived in typical suburban houses and cruised through town in cars that you see on any North American street.

Dennis Lee, who is in his late eighties, leads a fairly typical life in Loma Linda. I caught up to him when he had a few minutes of downtime, a rarity. Even though it was a day off from his job as a hospital pharmacist, Lee was busy. I'd just watched him participate in an hour-long, high-energy aerobics class open only to those sixty-five or older at the Loma Linda University's Drayton Center, a sprawling complex of exercise machines, weight rooms, gymnasiums, squash courts, tennis courts, and swimming pools. The facility seemed like overkill for a school with an enrollment of fewer than 4,500, but everything on offer was well used.

Just watching Lee and his three dozen companions sent my pulse rate up. To the deafening beat of "Y.M.C.A." and a nonstop stream of similar hits from the '70s and '80s, the class worked through frenetic sessions of jumping, running in place, stretching, floor exercises, routines with soccer ball–size medicine balls, and repetitive weight lifting. Instructor Sandy Bernier, a lean, spandex-clad dynamo, had scolded me half-jokingly when I sat in a chair on the sidelines of the workout room. "Sitting is the enemy," she said, grinning. Lee, a compact man who, despite his age, still had a full head of black hair, spoke to me during a few spare minutes between Bernier's class and a stint in the weight room, which preceded his half hour jogging on a treadmill. After that, he planned to unwind with a few ferocious sets of Ping-Pong and then head home to tend his expansive vegetable garden, a source of both fresh produce and outdoor exercise. He followed that same routine every day that he was not filling prescriptions and overseeing junior members at the pharmacy. Lee was far from the oldest participant in Bernier's Silver Fox class. When I asked him for the secret of his age-defying stamina, he gave a shy, awe-shucks-it's-nothin' grin and said, "I exercise a lot, I watch my eating, plus positive thinking."

To grab something quick for lunch after meeting with Lee, I stopped at the Loma Linda Market, a grocery store that at first glance could have been in any mall in America. But as soon as I entered, I found myself facing a "juicery" with a couple of hip young fellows pushing carrots, stacked on the counter like saw logs, into the rotating jaws of a crushing machine. Beyond the juicery, I encountered an entire aisle of plastic bulk containers of herbs, teas, and grains, an astounding number of which contained nuts and seeds. I could find no coffee—unless you counted a few shelves of chicory-based stuff, which should be an illegal substance in my caffeine-addicted opinion. I managed to spot two forlorn bottles of milk—the type that comes from a cow—tucked away in a back corner of a "dairy case." The bottles looked like the poor relatives of a colorful selection of cartons of milk substitutes made from almonds, coconuts, oats, and soy. I found a few dozen eggs, but not a single slice of meat or drop of beer or wine. As for cigarettes and other tobacco products, forget it. A city ordinance bans smoking in town, even outdoors (but you can light up on your own property). Later, when I inquired if a fellow could get a drink anywhere nearby, Briana Pastorino, a youngish public affairs officer for the hospital who appeared to be of an age where she would know the local action spots, told me that she thought there might be a few restaurants where you could get a beer or a glass of wine. But hard liquor? Definitely not. Given my experiences at the supermarket and the Drayton Center, I concluded that residents of Loma Linda would have to make a concerted effort to avoid exercising and eating healthy food.

The market did, however, have a large section set aside for books and magazines arranged in categories like Christian lifestyle and Seventh-day faith and heritage, in case I needed spiritual refreshment. I was reminded of a brief conversation I'd had earlier with Jennifer Sawyer, a pert, gray-haired woman behind the reception desk at the center where the aerobics class was held. I told her I'd come to Loma Linda hoping to discover a few tips on how the Adventists outlived most Americans. Although I did not ask her, Sawyer, who was in her seventies, was eager to give her opinion: "Portion control. Gratitude. Laughter. And mindfulness."

As I walked away, she called out, "And remember, God wants us to have an enjoyable time."

In the back of my mind, a skeptical little voice asked, "Okay, but does God really want me to eat stir-fried soy-based meat replacements?"

CHAPTER NINE

CLUB MED

During a cooking class that I attended at the home of Aglaia Kremezi, on the Greek island of Kea, she upended a full bottle of olive oil over a skillet filled with chopped onions. And kept it upended. It was the first time I'd seen her standing still all morning. Kremezi is a renowned expert on the foods of Greece, the author of several cookbooks, and one of the single most energetic humans I've encountered. With her auburn hair and youthful build, she could pass for forty, although I suspect she's a couple of decades older than that.

I had traveled to Kea to learn firsthand about the Mediterranean diet and the legendary health benefits it delivers. I can think of no better guide than Kremezi, who nonchalantly allowed the amber liquid to glug into the pan for so long that I was beginning to wonder if I was being made the butt of some culinary joke. Finally, she stopped pouring, nodded with satisfaction, and said the obvious: "In Greek cuisine, we use a lot of olive oil."

Good thing for the Kremezi family finances that a dozen olive trees sagged under a ripening load of fruit in their yard.

With the oil and onion mixture sizzling, Kremezi, her husband Costas Moraitis, her assistant, my wife, and I proceeded to prepare the rest of our lunch, a medley of stuffed tomatoes, stuffed bell peppers, and stuffed baby eggplants. With paring knives, we cut off and saved the tops, then hollowed out the vegetables until they looked like faceless, miniature jack-o'-lanterns and set them aside. We diced the "guts" of the tomatoes and eggplants, and added them to the onions, along with some chopped bell pepper, rice, pine nuts, raisins, farro (a variety of wheat), and handfuls of parsley, dill, mint, and oregano (Kremezi had foraged the mint and oregano, which grow wild on the island). Once softened, everything went into the hollowed vegetables, which were placed in a roasting pan and sealed with their original tops. After an hour in the oven, lunch was ready.

When I'd gone on Dean Ornish's low-fat, vegan diet, I often had difficulty feeling full. I would leave the table hungry and a little resentful after most meals; and well before it was time to eat again, I was positively famished. Maybe veganism wasn't for me? But that day, over a leisurely lunch in the shady bower that served as both a dining area and an outdoor extension of Kremezi's kitchen, I felt comfortably satiated, so much so that the best I could do was take a polite nibble of the beautiful branzino that Moraitis had flavored with thyme, basil, mint, and rosemary; wrapped in

MEDITERRANEAN DIET

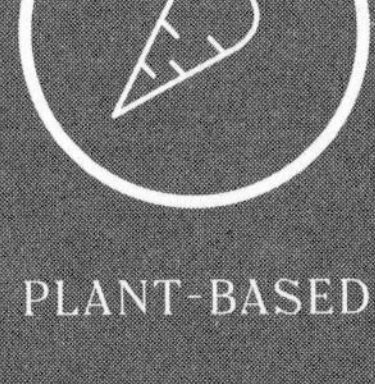

PLANT-BASED

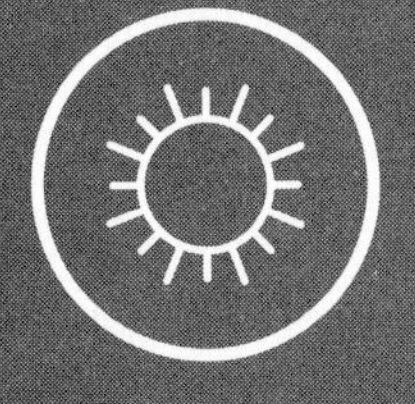

SEASONAL AND
LOCAL INGREDIENTS

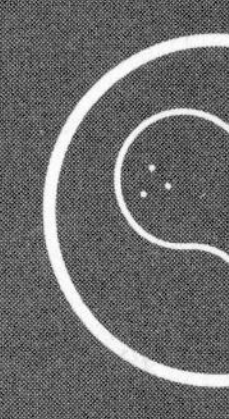

LIMITED MEAT
AND DAIRY

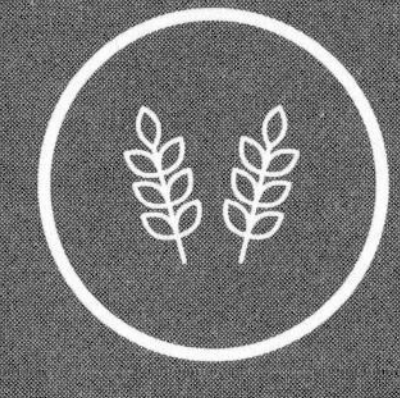

INCLUDES
AROMATIC HERBS

FAT INTAKE COMES
FROM OLIVE OIL

MODEST AMOUNT OF
WINE WITH MEALS

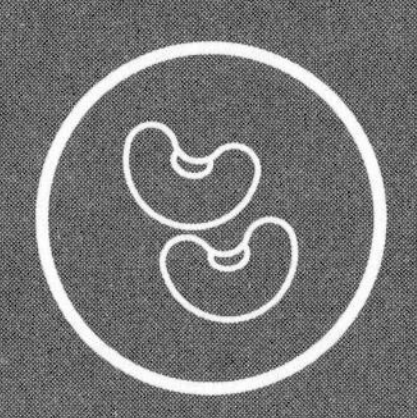

LOTS OF VEGETABLES,
FRUIT, LEGUMES, NUTS, AND
UNPROCESSED GRAINS

fig leaves (from a tree in their yard); and grilled over an open fire. I left the table full, but far from bloated, and had energy enough to spend a couple of hours that afternoon walking along the ancient donkey paths, which have become popular hiking trails on modern Kea. I wasn't particularly hungry when dinnertime came, so I contented myself with nibbling two savory barley biscuits, a specialty of the island.

And so my lunches on Kea went. Paper-thin layers of phyllo dough filled with horta, or wild greens, one afternoon. A puree of yellow split peas topped by wilted dandelion greens another day. An eggplant ragout on a third day. Each dish was well lubricated with olive oil, heavily accented by fresh herbs, and washed down with a glass of wine. Animal products—fish, squid, lamb, and a crumbly white cheese made from sheep's and goat's milk—played minor supporting roles. Aside from a small bowl of yogurt for breakfast, not a single product from a cow passed my lips. "You cook with the vegetables you have," Kremezi said. "The olive oil and the herbs make you feel satisfied."

I can't remember many trips when I've eaten so well, and none when I returned weighing three pounds less than I did when I set out.

That visit confirmed everything I'd learned about the benefits of the so-called Mediterranean diet. One massive study launched in 1993 has followed more than 28,000 Greek men. Those who eat traditional fare have lower rates of heart disease, cancer, diabetes, stroke, and overall mortality than comparable groups in eight other European countries. The diet was also found to promote weight loss in obese subjects and prevent those who were not obese from becoming so. A 2013 paper showed that adopting a Mediterranean diet could stop 30 percent of heart attacks and strokes. It seems counterintuitive, but the diet delivers all these benefits even as it derives a whopping 40 percent of its calories from fat, substantially higher than the average American diet, which is about 35 percent fat. Yet Americans are heavier and less healthy. The key difference is that most of the fat in the Greek diet comes from olive oil. We Americans get more of our fat from red meat, butter, and other animal products.

Despite being plant based, the Mediterranean diet does not dogmatically eliminate any of the major food groups and does not require carefully measuring every morsel destined for your plate. Greeks just eat. Period. According to Dr. Dariush Mozaffarian, head of the Freidman School of Nutrition Science and Policy at Tufts University, Greeks stay healthy while ignoring calories, portion sizes, and specific nutrients. It is the overall quality of their diet that keeps their rate of obesity low.

Moreover, the traditional Greek diet has stood the test of time—it's the opposite of a fad diet. Many of the dishes I enjoyed in Kremezi's shady dining area appear in nearly identical form in the comical plays of Aristophanes, which were performed 2,500 years ago and in which eating was a prominent theme. Archaeological evidence points to even earlier origins. The Greeks ate food that came from the ingredients provided by the region's scant summer rainfall and thin soils: greens, fruits, legumes, barley, and small amounts of meat. And many citizens still do. Seafood, never a major source of calories, came from local waters.

The Mediterranean diet's transition from meager fare that had sustained peasants for millennia into the darling of modern cookbook authors and nutrition experts owes a great deal to a group of ambitious researchers and clever marketers. In the second half of the twentieth century, they harnessed the power of the media to promote paradigm-changing dietary research. First and foremost among those was a University of Minnesota scientist named Ancel Keys, whose career was distinguished, varied, and, at times, controversial.

During World War II, he concocted the formula for the famous K rations (*K* as in Keys), easily carried food packets that would not spoil and supplied enough energy to sustain American soldiers. At a time when millions of Europeans faced famine due to the deprivations of war, Keys also oversaw the ominously named Minnesota Starvation Study, which involved putting a group of subjects on an extreme low-calorie regimen to examine the effects of near-starvation, and tracking their subsequent weight gain when they began eating normal quantities again. But it was his theory about the relationship between consuming saturated fat and developing heart disease that ensured his status as one of the twentieth century's most influential nutrition researchers. Keys' work popularized the gospel of a diet low in saturated fat, which came to dominate dietary recommendations.

Brilliant, blunt, and intellectually pugilistic, Keys also oversaw the seminal Seven Countries Study. Beginning in 1958, he and his associates tracked the health of more than twelve thousand men in the United States, Italy, Finland, the Netherlands, Japan, Greece, and the country then called Yugoslavia. Before the study, the onset of heart disease was generally viewed as an inevitable function of aging, like gray hair and wrinkled skin. Nothing could be done to prevent it. But examinations of men on the Greek islands of Corfu and Crete shortly after World War II showed remarkably low levels of coronary disease, and the men often continued hard manual labor well into their nineties (and still enjoyed regular sex) at a time when much younger and more well-to-do Americans were clutching their chests and keeling over from heart attacks.

Keys thought diet might explain the difference. He had selected the seven countries because of the dramatic disparities between their populations' consumption of saturated fat. Tabulated and published between 1966 and 1986, the results showed that groups who ate large amounts of saturated fat, like those studied in the United States and Finland, had rates of heart disease as much as ten times higher than those living in countries bordering the Mediterranean. The hard-scrabble farmers of Corfu and Crete were among the healthiest of all. Keys became a confirmed advocate for the Mediterranean way of eating and popularized his work in books such as the 1975 bestseller, *How to Eat Well and Stay Well the Mediterranean Way*. Keys' own life lent validity to his scientific conclusions. He remained intellectually active until his late nineties and passed away a few weeks before he would have turned 101 years old.

Keys may be the father of the Mediterranean diet as we now understand it. The woman recognized throughout the nutrition community as its mother is Antonia Trichopoulou, a medical doctor who is president of the nonprofit Hellenic Health Foundation in Athens and holds positions at the University of Athens Medical School and the World Health Organization—jobs with responsibilities that make for a full workweek, especially for someone in her eighties. In the mid-1980s, she became convinced that her homeland's foodways had both culinary and health benefits. This was at a time when Greeks, influenced by American scientists' focus on corn, soybean, and other vegetable oils commonly available in the United States, were cutting back on their use of olive oil. Greek farmers had even begun razing groves of olive trees.

For a while, Trichopoulou followed the prevailing trend away from olive oil by encouraging the cooks at the hospitals she advised to switch to vegetable oils. But she had little success. ("I can't cook without olive oil," one cafeteria manager complained.) Trichopoulou ultimately realized that trying to change ingrained culinary customs was a fool's errand and might produce negative health effects. "Tradition rarely honors unhealthy habits," she told me. She began to fight for her country's cuisine, organizing and presiding over a series of academic conferences to bring the attention of the world's leading nutritionists to the benefits of the Mediterranean diet. Over the decades, Trichopoulou has authored scores of scientific papers on its health benefits and accumulated a collection of two hundred authentic traditional recipes from remote regions of the country.

Her efforts caught the attention of a Boston-based organization, Oldways Preservation Trust, which was dedicated to preserving heritage foods, ingredients, and culinary practices. Beginning in the early 1990s, Oldways started offering food journalists and researchers fully paid junkets funded by the olive oil industry to areas where the traditional Mediterranean diet survived. The pampered and well-fed writers dutifully returned home to sing the praises of the healthful foods of these beautiful, sun-drenched regions.

After leaving Kea, I visited Trichopoulou at her summer home on the coast about forty-five minutes south of Athens. She invited me to join her on the balcony, which opened onto a scene that seemed to come right out of a promotional brochure from the Greek tourism office. The sea, choppy and cobalt blue, lapped a beach below us. Traditional, high-bowed fishing caïques put-putted across the harbor, mingling incongruously with sleek recreational yachts and their billowing white sails. Dun-colored mountains provided a jagged backdrop, and there wasn't a cloud in the sky. It struck me, not for the first time, that the reason Greeks enjoy such longevity might have as much to do with where they live as with what they eat. If I were fortunate enough to pass my days on places such as Trichopoulou's balcony and Kremezi's yard, with its fig, almond, citrus, and olive trees, I would do everything in my power to savor life for as long as possible.

Snacking from a bowl of bright-red pomegranate seeds, Trichopoulou, who wore a flowery summer dress, was charming and occasionally mischievous—until our small talk ended and our discussion turned to her work, at which point she became direct and businesslike. I first wanted to clear up something that had confused me. What, exactly, did she mean when she used the term *Mediterranean diet*? After all, nations as diverse as Israel, Egypt, Morocco, Spain, France, Italy, and Greece all border the Mediterranean, and their cuisines are vastly different.

"In my work, I am very strict on the definition of the Mediterranean diet," she said. "When we speak of its health benefits, we are talking about those parts of the Mediterranean basin where olive trees grow and how the people living there ate before 1960. It is characterized by high consumption of vegetables, fruits, legumes, nuts, and unprocessed grains, and low consumption of meat and dairy products. Moderate consumption of wine with meals is also a trait."

I also asked her to explain what I'd come to think of as the Greek paradox—how any diet that derives 40 percent of its calories from fat could be healthful. Trichopoulou explained that she prefers to use the term *so-called fat*, when referring to olive oil, because to northern Europeans and Americans *fat* means one thing: animal fat. To southern Europeans *fat* means olive oil. "Fats and oils are distinct categories in the broader group of lipids," she said.

A 2006 study conducted by researchers in Spain corroborated the unique properties of olive oil. It examined more than seven thousand university students and concluded, "A high amount of olive oil consumption is not associated with higher weight gain or a significantly higher risk of developing overweight or obesity in the context of the Mediterranean food plan." Being unsaturated, meaning that it is liquid at room temperature, olive oil has been found to be more heart healthful than the saturated fat in animal products such as meat, lard, and butter, which are solid at room temperature.

Despite olive oil's health benefits, Trichopoulou cautioned me not to focus on any individual food or nutrient—including olive oil—as the key to the healthfulness of the Greek diet. "The combination of different foods might be essential to get the effect, not single components," she said. "There could be interactions among different foods."

All those vegetables and herbs that Kremezi taught me how to prepare might also be playing a key role in keeping Greeks healthy. According to a 2005 study that Trichopoulou co-authored, vegetables, seeds, and legumes are good sources of flavonoids, powerful antioxidants that help prevent or slow cancer and heart disease. The ever-present herbs and spices in Greek dishes are also filled with flavonoids. The typical Greek diet has about 50 percent more of these protective plant chemicals than the U.S. diet. Even those sweet pomegranate seeds Trichopoulou and I snacked on during our interview were loaded with antioxidants.

Olive oil also contains high amounts of those beneficial compounds—much higher than oils derived from corn, rape seeds (commonly called canola oil), or soybeans. Such seed oils are manufactured using chemical solvents, which greatly reduce the seeds' quantities of protective compounds. Olive oil, on the other hand, is simply pressed out of the olives. It receives no further treatment, ensuring that it retains the original antioxidants. Of course, olive oil has another big advantage: great taste, which makes fresh herbs and greens even more alluring.

One other ever-present component of the country's cuisine might also contribute to Greeks' health. No lunch or dinner there is complete without wine. According to Trichopoulou, evidence suggests that wine, particularly red wine, is not only high in antioxidants itself but may also help the body absorb nutrients when consumed with olive oil in the same meal. However, she added an immediate caveat: Most Greeks drink only small amounts of wine. Men typically consume no

MEDITERRANEAN DIET STATS

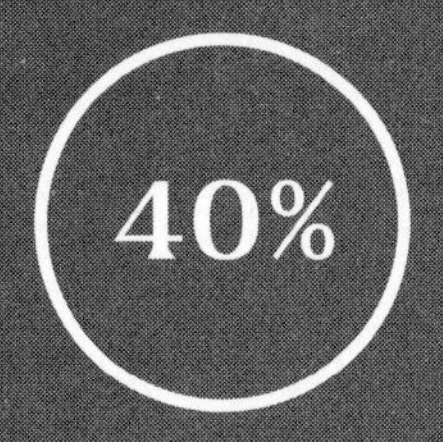

CALORIES FROM FAT

VERSUS

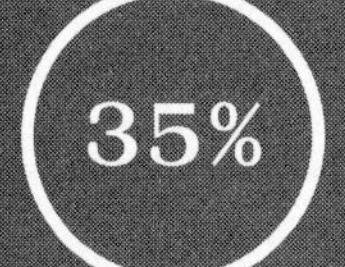

AVERAGE AMERICAN DIET

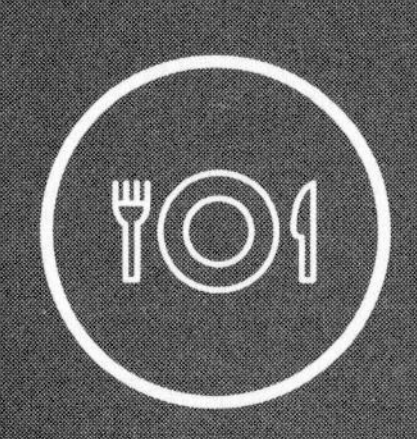

THE TYPICAL GREEK DIET HAS 50% MORE PROTECTIVE PLANT COMPOUNDS IN IT THAN THE TYPICAL AMERICAN DIET.

GREEK MEN WHO EAT THE TRADITIONAL DIET HAVE DECREASED RATES OF HEART DISEASE, CANCER, DIABETES, AND STROKE THAN SIMILAR GROUPS IN EIGHT OTHER EUROPEAN COUNTRIES.

ADOPTING A MEDITERRANEAN DIET HAS BEEN SHOWN TO REDUCE THE RISK OF HEART ATTACKS AND STROKES BY 30%.

more than a couple of glasses per day, women maybe one, and always with a meal.

Among Greeks today, Trichopoulou said, adherence to the traditional diet is unfortunately in decline. The drop has provided something of a real-life experiment. Although heart disease remains relatively low in Greece, it is not dropping, whereas other European countries are experiencing a drop. "Why?" she asked, rhetorically. "First, we no longer have time to cook at home the traditional way. It's quick and easy to get a steak and fries on the table. People are forsaking wine for whiskey and beer, which they consume outside of meals. In the past, there was no binging. That is changing. White bread has replaced dark bread." Moreover, the younger generation has all but abandoned the traditional diet, gulping soda and gobbling sugary snacks with the same abandon as teenagers in the rest of the developed world.

Supporting Trichopoulou's observation, one Italian study found that two-thirds of participants between the ages of fifteen and twenty-four said they no longer ate a Mediterranean diet. Trichopoulou suspects similar results would be found in Greece. Among European countries, Greece now has one of the highest rates of childhood obesity.

Given that I was about to return to my home in New England, I wondered whether it was possible for someone living in the United States to get the benefits of the traditional Greek diet. "Sure," Trichopoulou said without hesitation. "The Mediterranean diet is plant based. Respect that principle. It also uses seasonal and local ingredients. Do that, too, when you can. Start learning to cook with vegetables, and use lots of different kinds. If you prepare them with olive oil and add plenty of aromatic herbs, lemon, onions, and garlic, they make a good main dish. Don't forget legumes and fresh fruits. And remember, above all, the Mediterranean diet is successful because it calls for no willpower or sacrifice. People truly enjoy eating it."

CHAPTER TEN

A FRENCH CONNECTION

One version of Utopia for me would be a place where I could indulge in whatever foods I fancied, paying not the slightest regard to fattening calories and artery-clogging cholesterol. I'd eat marbled steaks with french fries, chicken breasts smothered with decadent sauces, and sole fillets sautéed in butter—wonderful, rich, golden butter. If I fancied a schmear of triple-crème cheese or a wedge of a tangy blue, along with a piece of bread, no problem. I could indulge in foie gras or duck confit at will, and breakfast on fluffy omelets. Some of the greatest wines would enhance the pleasure of dining. And, best of all, my chances of growing fat or having a heart attack would be far lower than they are in the world where I wage a daily battle against excess weight.

Such a place exists. It's called France.

Somehow, the French consume some of the tastiest food in the world, deriving an average of nearly 40 percent of their calories from fat. And unlike the Greek diet, which is identically as high in fat, the French diet is high in saturated fat. Still, the French maintain low rates of obesity and cardiovascular disease. While four in ten Americans rate as clinically obese, less than half that portion of French people are similarly robust. A resident of France is 60 percent less likely to die of circulatory disease (including heart attacks) than someone living in the United States. The French spend more time eating than do residents of any other developed country, and yet they stay thin—much thinner on average than Americans. It's called the French paradox, and whatever name you call it by, it just doesn't seem fair. In my quest for a better physique, maybe I could learn a thing or two from the French.

Jacques Pépin, a French chef who came to the United States in 1959 and stayed to build a career as a well-known author, teacher, and television personality, introduced me to that paradox when I assisted him with a book project in the early 2000s. To work with Pépin is to eat with him, and whether our sessions were held in his Manhattan office at the International Culinary Center, where he was a dean, or at his Connecticut home, lunch inevitably followed. A very good lunch.

I suspect it was no coincidence that Pépin's friends and business associates had a habit of dropping by around the noon hour. No meal at his house started without a basket of bread and a bottle of wine on the table. Pépin effortlessly conjured up delicious dishes, often from leftovers in his fridge: a stew of pork kidneys, lamb tongue, and navy beans (scrumptious, believe me); slivers of fatty smoked duck breast; or homemade sausages gifted to him by a friend. No meal ended without a plate of two or three cheeses passed around the table. And these were quick, working lunches. Pépin is in his mid-eighties and still going strong. He carries a small, well-earned paunch but is spry and far from obese. "I am not overweight," he agreed, with a self-deprecating smile. He patted his stomach. "Well, perhaps a bit under-tall."

Although he is rightly famous as a culinary instructor, on this occasion, I was visiting him to learn some lessons on the proper way to eat, not cook. How do the French do it? Or more to the point, how does Pépin continue to do it after more than six decades in this country—half a world and an unbridgeable cultural gulf away from the town in southeastern France where he grew up?

Pépin was born with a hearty appetite and a pitch-perfect palate. But he is the opposite of a food snob, and despite working in the legendary bastions of haute cuisine in Paris and as the personal chef to French President Charles de Gaulle, he has taken to the foods of his adopted country with egalitarian gusto. After a stint at New York's posh Le Pavillon, at the time the most renowned French restaurant in this country, he passed up an offer to become the White House chef for the Kennedys (been there, done that). Instead he cheerfully rolled up his sleeves behind the grill of a remote Howard Johnson's outpost in Queens, because he was eager to understand Americans' eating habits. Today he's as likely to slap a rack of spareribs on his grill or throw together a Cuban casserole of black beans as he is to cook coq au vin. But while his appetite is unabashedly Americanized, his philosophy on dining has remained steadfastly French. "I have absolutely no guilty food sins," he said. "I always eat with pleasure and no guilt."

One thing Pépin has never done is go on a diet. "If I overdo it, I'll cut back for a day or two—but I eat what I would normally eat, I never avoid a specific food," he said. In our meals together, Pépin partook of everything, but he refrained from seconds.

He and his wife, Gloria, who has a physique that sets the standard for birdlike, have been married for more than fifty years, and he can't remember an evening at home when they haven't sat down together for dinner—no eating on the run or gobbling something quick while standing at the kitchen island. Even on weeknights with just two of them in the house, the meal begins with bread and wine, which are followed by three or four small dishes, consumed leisurely over the course of an hour. Dessert is usually a selection of pungent cheeses or a simple preparation showcasing whatever fruit is at the height of ripeness. The night before I dropped by, he and Gloria had dined on grilled quail, grilled portobello mushrooms, corn on the cob, and a green salad. They ended the meal with slices of Comté cheese. "We each had a morsel of the cheese, a taste—about the size of a domino," he said. "If you eat slower and eat better, taking the time to taste what you put in your mouth, you eat less and enjoy it more. You get satisfied. One of the biggest things in the way the French dine is that we have smaller portions. I'll never forget the first time my mother, who loved roast beef, came over to visit. We took her to a restaurant, and when she saw the size of her prime rib, she nearly fell off her chair. She thought it was for the entire table of eight."

Pépin is convinced that choosing the best-tasting food available contributes to weight maintenance and overall health, whether it's seasonal fruits and vegetables, pastured eggs, or even expensive Kobe beef, which he described as wonderful. "Three ounces are enough to satisfy anyone. On the other hand, you can eat and eat and yet never feel satisfied if you consume poor-quality food." That is especially true for processed and packaged food, which he completely avoids.

Sitting down and enjoying a meal without distractions is an inviolate rule chez Pépin. "When you don't take time to eat," he states "when you grab a sandwich or something, an hour later you won't even remember what you have eaten—it's the same if you eat while reading the paper, or looking at an iPhone, or walking down the street. The function of having eaten almost ceases to exist in your mind because it gets overshadowed. There are people who eat ten times a day and never sit down to dinner. And they get fat."

Food is, above all, improved by the simple act of being shared. "I recently went to someone's home and saw the father eating while watching TV." "In another room, a kid was on his computer with a plate beside it. The mother was somewhere else. It was suppertime, and they were all over the house. It depressed me. I don't remember our daughter, Claudine, ever eating alone when she was young. Cooking and eating together is a way to communicate with kids—it's communal."

The value of sitting around a table cannot be underestimated. According to Pépin, "Wars have been avoided over a meal. People fall in love. The table is a sacred place."

It turns out that much of what Pépin told me anecdotally has the backing of solid academic studies. French citizens may look like us and enjoy similar developed-world standards of living, but when it comes to food, the attitudes between our two cultures could hardly be more divergent. In the book *Manger* ("To Eat"), Claude Fischler, a sociologist and anthropologist at the French National Center for Scientific Research, catalogs the results of a series of surveys conducted between 2000 and 2002 in Paris and Philadelphia that compared how the French and Americans view the act of eating.

According to Fischler's results, the French people he surveyed, similar to Pépin, tended to see eating as inexorably linked to ritual and sociability—to community in the broadest sense. Americans, conversely, viewed eating as a biological function best dealt with as efficiently and rapidly as possible. The French adhere to clearly established mealtimes,

FRENCH VERSUS AMERICAN APPROACH TO EATING

FRENCH

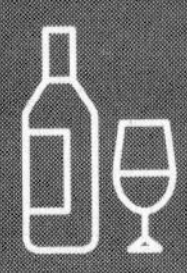

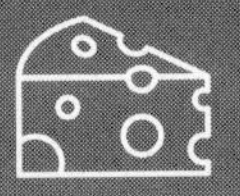

QUALITY JOY RITUAL

COMMUNITY SELECTION

AMERICAN

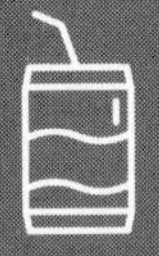

QUANTITY ABUNDANCE INDIVIDUAL

BIOLOGICAL COMFORT

during which they enjoy food and converse with companions. They can't conceive of "eating well" unless it is in the context of being together with associates, friends, or loved ones. Americans see nothing wrong with working or performing other tasks while eating, as if time spent at the table is somehow wasted. The French view our cavalier attitude toward eating as barbaric and animal-like, while we find the French rigidity and formality to run contrary to our spirit of individualism and democratic principles. Fischler concludes that their emphasis on community plays a major role in protecting the French from becoming obese.

The Americans he surveyed regarded food as a form of medicine and tended to focus on calories or on the health benefits or drawbacks of single nutrients. ("You should eat blueberries for their antioxidants." "Oranges are high in vitamin C.") Like Pépin, the French focus on quality and on what Fischler calls the identity of food products—terroir and authenticity. They eat a cuisine. Americans focus on individual foods and tend to view them in terms of what they *don't* have: no cholesterol, no fat, no gluten, no sugar. The French associate food with pleasure. Nonetheless, they are far more convinced than Americans that what they eat is healthful.

Because of our emphasis on individualism, Americans put far more value on having a wide number of mealtime choices than do the French. Fischler presented groups of French and American subjects with the following scenario: You want some ice cream. You have the choice between two ice-cream parlors. The first offers fifty different flavors. The second only ten. Assuming the prices are equal, which would you chose? Among Americans, 56 percent opted for the fifty-flavor establishment, compared to only 32 percent of the French. Fischler speculates that while the French are willing to accept that the owner of the ten-flavor scoop shop selects his limited inventory with care and on the basis of quality, Americans prefer a large number of choices to make their own individual decisions. Pépin—no surprise—is typically French. "If I have a choice between two restaurants, one with forty items on the menu, the other with five, I will choose the one with five. I know what cooks can do, and it would be impossible for most to master forty dishes. With five, the chef will be focusing on what he does best." In France, tradition trumps individualism. The French know with certainty that steak must be accompanied by *frites*—french fries. When ordering a steak, Americans prefer the choice of having their potatoes mashed, baked, or fried.

Harvey Levenstein, an emeritus professor of history at Ontario's McMaster University, has focused much of his research on North America's culinary traditions, or lack thereof. English immigrants to the United States were constrained by a strong Protestant ethic, which made them feel guilty about eating too well, according to Levenstein. "People felt they had to control their consumption of food," he told me. The same Protestant ethic instilled a deep suspicion of pleasure. "Self-denial leads to good things. Self-indulgence leads to bad things. That is the essence of New England Protestantism—and the country's early home economists were all New England Protestants. Think of the lasting influence of the *Boston Cooking School Cookbook* by Fannie Farmer, which was published in the late 1800s. They were all uptight. You don't find the same thing in the cuisines of Catholic countries."

Paul Rozin, a psychologist at the University of Pennsylvania, who has partnered with Claude Fischler in several studies, agrees. During a phone call with me, he said part of the explanation for the fundamental difference in French and American attitudes toward eating can be traced to the historical role of Catholicism, which emphasizes community, versus Protestantism, which focuses on individual responsibility.

Rozin has determined that Americans prefer what he calls comforts, things that make life easier. The French opt instead for joys, unique

A FRENCH RECIPE

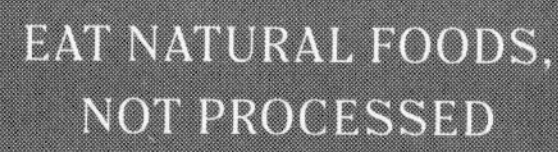

EAT NATURAL FOODS,
NOT PROCESSED

EAT AT THE TABLE

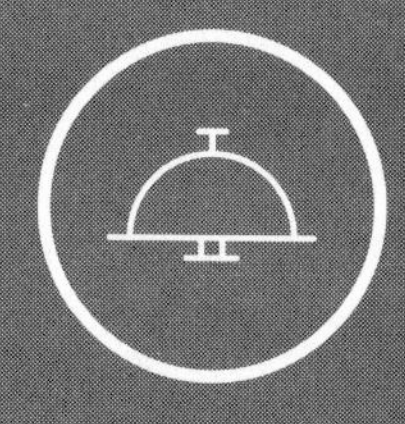

EAT THE BEST
QUALITY FOODS

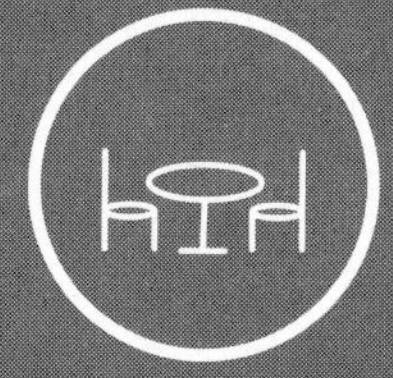

MAKE EATING
COMMUNAL

EAT SENSIBLE
PORTIONS

EAT ALL FOODS
IN MODERATION

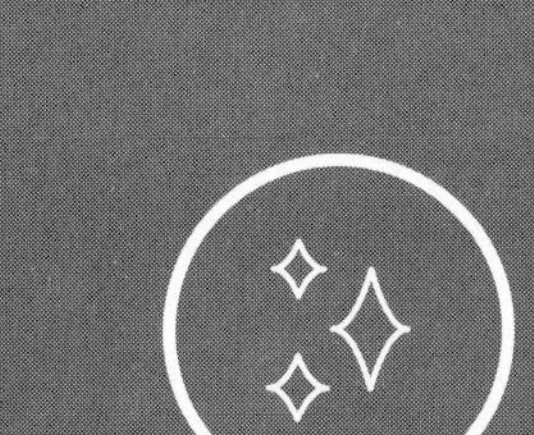

UPHOLD JOY
OVER COMFORT

experiences that make life interesting. Americans' preference of quantity over quality comes from our ingrained focus on abundance. From the early days of European settlement on this continent, visitors marveled at the huge amount of food colonists had to eat. It's no coincidence that Thanksgiving, our national holiday, is dedicated to stuffing ourselves—a sharp contrast to the French preference for moderation.

The result of their emphasis on quality over quantity is that French define good food as elegant, sophisticated, and attractively presented, standards they inherited from the country's early gastronomes, who also emphasized the value of moderation. "Because of that, French portions are notably smaller than American portion sizes," Rozin said. He suggested that one simple, practical way to close the obesity gap between the two cultures would be for American cooks to offer smaller portions. "People eat what they are served," he said.

"American cuisine has no specific flavor profile," according to Rozin. "That's because we've always eaten a lot of meat here. Meat is flavorful in and of itself, so you don't have to worry about adding flavor with a palate of spices." This lack of culinary traditions to fall back upon, which the French, Greeks, Mexicans, Indians, Vietnamese, Japanese, and many other cultures have in abundance, is bad for our health. It makes us seek out simple solutions. Americans, he said, tend to divide food into two distinct categories—healthful versus unhealthful. We see food and disease as part of the same continuum. The French, on the other hand, separate food from health and disease. They divide what they eat into the categories of natural versus processed.

In contrast to Pépin, who maintained his Gallic approach to the table when he came to the United States, Mireille Guiliano abandoned hers when she made the same journey at age eighteen as an exchange student in the late 1960s. She ate like her new American classmates, and the result was predictable: she packed on fifteen pounds during the school year, enough to make her father greet her upon her return home with the words, "You look like a sack of potatoes."

Guiliano soon banished those excess pounds and ultimately put the experience to good use by parlaying what she learned from her year of plumpness and subsequent weight loss into the 2005 bestseller *French Women Don't Get Fat*. Although the book drew criticism for sexist stereotyping, Guiliano, who returned to the United States as head of American operations for champagne maker Veuve Clicquot, does provide what amounts to a manual about how Americans can put the research by Fischler, Rozin, and other academics to practical use. Despite the title of her book, her advice applies equally to overweight American women and men.

"Eating in America has become controversial behavior, with all sorts of 'nonnutritional,' sexual, social, political, cultural, and even clinical overtones," Guiliano writes. "Our troubles with weight have as much to do with our attitudes toward eating as they do with what we are ingesting. We are seeing a growing psychosis that I believe actually adds stress to our already stressful way of life. It is fast erasing the simple values of pleasure. Without a national change of heart, we have little hope of turning back the tide of obesity."

That change of heart would involve observing some straightforward rules that Guiliano sets out:

- → Eat smaller portions of more things.
- → Eat all things, but in moderation.
- → Eat lots of fruits and vegetables.
- → Eat with all your senses.

- → Eat three meals a day.
- → Don't snack.
- → Don't eat until you feel stuffed, but don't let yourself leave the table hungry.
- → Honor mealtime and don't eat on the run, standing, or in front of a TV.
- → Eat seasonally for maximum flavor.
- → Enjoy wine, by all means, but a glass or two at most and only with meals.

Guiliano was finally able to drop and permanently keep off the "sack of potatoes" pounds she gained as a student when, at the advice of her family doctor in France, she learned to identify and limit, or temporarily abolish, key food offenders, which she sometimes calls, with a nod to the film *Casablanca*, "the usual suspects." If any of these offenders (in her case, pastries) regularly appear on your menu, Guiliano says you should view it as an opportunity. There is only one way to find these culprits, she says: use your own intuition.

CHAPTER ELEVEN

THE RECKONING

It's never a good thing when your doctor calls you unexpectedly at 7:15 a.m. on a Friday morning.

Because of my family's history of coronary disease, Doctor Dennis and I had been closely monitoring my heart for years. We scrupulously tracked my cholesterol levels and blood pressure. I'd had numerous electrocardiograms and once underwent a cardiac stress test. Technicians had me run on a treadmill until I reached a point of near exhaustion, after which they did a nuclear scan of the vessels supplying my heart to see if any blockages impeded blood flow.

I had passed all the tests, if not with flying colors, then at least with acceptable results. But I'd never had a coronary calcium test to measure the level of plaque in my arteries. Like high cholesterol and high blood pressure, having high amounts of plaque is an indicator of the possibility of a cardiac event. As plaque builds, it can rupture, creating a blood clot. If the clot clogs a coronary artery, the section of heart muscle the artery supplies becomes starved of oxygen and dies, resulting in a heart attack. After Arthur Agatston had so emphatically recommended the procedure when I visited him in South Beach, I asked Doctor Dennis to schedule one for me. It might have saved my life.

The results of the scan explained the early-morning call. They'd just come in, and they were terrible. My calcium level was in the ninetieth percentile for men my age—and this is one test where the last thing you want is to be at the top of the class. Doctor Dennis made an appointment for me to see a cardiologist as soon as possible.

That call set the stage for the glummest Easter weekend I have ever experienced. My wife and I planned to spend Friday and Saturday nights in New York City, where we would take in a play and eat lots of good food. We'd get back home on Sunday in time to host a big holiday dinner for the entire family, who, for once, were going to be in the same place at the same time.

We went ahead with our plans to go to the city, but I could not get my mind off those test results. At Grand Central Oyster Bar, I've always loved the classic (if decadent) oyster pan roast, a house specialty featuring oysters swimming in a bowl filled to the rim with Heinz chili sauce and enormous quantities of half-and-half atop a slab of white toast. The prospect of adding even more plaque to my arteries demolished my appetite for that dish. Instead, I opted for a broiled Arctic char fillet and skipped the two glasses of wine I would have had on a typical evening out. Doctor Dennis's news cast a pall over the Easter table, too. I took only a thin slice of our traditional ham, carefully carving away any visible traces of fat. My wife and kids were worried about me, and I felt guilty, as if it were my fault that no one felt festive.

I was a failure. I'd been on The Whole30, Ornish's diet, South Beach, Atkins, paleo, Weight Watchers, and others. I'd been a vegetarian and a vegan. I'd cleansed and gone gluten free. I thought I had become more vigilant about what I was eating and was exercising. The banality of the results depressed me. Just as everything I had heard and read foretold, I am a world champion at shedding 5 to 10 percent of my body weight during formal diet regimes—then gaining every ounce back. What was a food-loving guy to do? Move to Loma Linda? France? Greece? It was time to take a hard look at what I ate and drank, and ruthlessly weed out Guiliano's "usual suspects." Spurred by my dreadful calcium score, I was determined to reassess my eating and make every change I could to lose weight and reduce my chances of having a heart attack. That meant confronting these offenders and banishing as many as I could, while relegating others to the status of very rare transgressions.

Although they disagreed on much, none of the experts I'd talked to—Ornish, Agatston, Fraser, Foster, Trichopoulou—had anything good to say about certain elements of the developed world's diet. Dr. David Ludwig, of Harvard Medical School, author of the book *Always Hungry? Conquer Cravings, Retrain Your Fat Cells, and Lose Weight Permanently*, doesn't hesitate to say that some foods are simply bad. "The argument that there are no bad foods reflects an obsolete nutrition paradigm and the food industry agenda, not the latest science," he told me. "Think of cigarettes. Taking a single puff is not going to kill you, yet no one today would hesitate about calling them bad. Well, some components of our diet are causing more illnesses and deaths than tobacco."

There is just one problem with the accepted wisdom that the only way to lose weight is to either eat less or move more—or both. "It doesn't work—not for most people over the long term," Ludwig said. In Ludwig's view, I may have fallen victim to what I call the Great Calorie Misconception. Many diet experts, Ludwig states, cling to the notion that a calorie is simply a calorie, a belief that hasn't changed since the 1800s when bloodletting was still considered to be the cure for nearly every ailment. In his view, the result has been catastrophic. "Obesity rates remain at historic highs, despite an incessant focus on calorie balance by the government, professional health associations, and the food industry," he reiterates.

Ludwig contends that, much like sugar, the processed carbs found in foods like white bread, white rice, and other baked goods are bad actors that pack fat onto our bodies in amounts that cannot be explained by their calorie content alone. "Conversely, nuts, olive oil, and dark chocolate—some of the most calorie-dense foods in existence—appear to prevent obesity, diabetes, and heart disease," he told me.

From a weight-loss point of view, is a Boston cream donut (270 calories at Dunkin') a better choice for breakfast than an egg and cheese sandwich on an English muffin, which has more calories (340)? For the last century and even longer, many food scientists, in effect, have responded with a resounding *yes*. In their thinking, the math is neat and in compliance with the first law of thermodynamics. The energy in that egg sandwich or donut will either be burned as fuel to keep you functioning or stored as fat. If you consume more calories than you expend, you gain weight. End of story. To lose weight, then, you must consume fewer calories than your body burns by eating less, or burn more calories than you consume by exercising more. Simple logic. Tough to argue with. But ask yourself this question: Do you really believe in your heart of hearts that, from a weight-loss standpoint, eating 100 calories of an egg and some cheese has the same effect as eating 100 calories of donut? Viewed in that light, the calorie-in calorie-out rule doesn't seem quite so logical. Ludwig says that we should forget calories.

It turns out that some of the components of our diet that affect weight gain cannot be explained by counting calories alone. These bad actors—sugar, processed carbohydrates, and alcohol—have insidious ways of forcing us to consume more calories than other foods. They do so by disrupting the mechanisms, both metabolic and mental, that tell us we've had enough to eat. They also create conditions that cause our bodies to store more of those calories as fat, rather than using them for energy.

In the United States, Canada, the United Kingdom, Australia, and other economically advanced countries, processed foods now account for half, or more, of calories consumed. "In the U.S., absolute intakes of protein and fat have remained relatively unchanged since the 1970s," said Ludwig. "Whereas carbohydrate (particularly refined grains, potato products, and added sugars) have increased markedly." The time frame coincides with the epidemic of obesity, and there's abundant evidence that processed carbs are a major culprit.

Demonstrating that all calories aren't created equal, Ludwig led a study of two groups of young adults who consumed diets containing the same number of calories. One group received meals high in refined carbohydrates, and the other ate low-carb meals. Despite consuming exactly the same number of calories, the low-carb contingent burned 325 calories per day more than their counterparts, an amount equal to an hour spent jogging or attending a yoga class. The low-carb food, Ludwig concluded, created conditions that made the body do a much better job of using the calories for energy, rather than stashing them away as fat.

According to Ludwig, refined starchy foods act in ways similar to sugar. They make blood glucose levels soar. This causes the pancreas to excrete more insulin, which in turn encourages fat cells to hoard calories. With that energy locked away in fat, there is too little fuel circulating to power the rest of the body, which then goes into what Ludwig calls the starvation response. Reacting as if you were truly starving, your metabolism slows to conserve energy, and your brain does everything it can to acquire more energy by encouraging you to eat more.

One of Ludwig's experiments clearly shows the starvation response in action. A group of adolescent boys ate different breakfasts on two mornings. On one, they dined on highly processed instant oatmeal. On the next, they ate vegetable omelets. Importantly, each meal contained precisely the same number of calories. Tests showed that the subjects' blood glucose levels started crashing about an hour after the oatmeal breakfast, driven by high insulin levels. After a few hours, adrenaline, a hormone excreted in response to stress, surged. The boys' brains thought they were having an energy crisis. On each day, a few hours after they'd had breakfast, the boys were given free access to all they could eat from a tasty buffet of bread, bagels, cream cheese, cheese spread, cold cuts, cookies, and fruit. After having processed oatmeal, the boys consumed 650 calories more from that buffet than after they had omelets, even though both breakfasts contained the same number of calories. "Because whole foods tend to digest slowly, some of their nutrients travel down the full length of the small intestines, stimulating powerful hormones that rev up metabolism and help us feel full," Ludwig explained. "Highly processed industrial foods digest in the first segments of the small intestine too quickly to trigger this built-in weight-regulating system."

Refined carbohydrates could have one other particularly malign effect on anyone trying to summon the willpower to avoid them. You may be hooked. Several recent studies have shown that so-called hyperpalatable foods such as french fries, pizza, and potato chips activate the same brain pathways as addictive drugs. In the journal *Medical Hypotheses*, Joan Ifland of the Refined Food Addiction Research Foundation, in Houston, writes, "The observational and empirical data strengthen the hypothesis that certain refined food consumption behaviors meet the criteria for substance abuse disorders." Like drug addicts, some people become refined-food junkies.

The irony, according to Ludwig, is that humans need to consume some protein and fat to survive but *can* get along eating no carbohydrates of any sort. Think of the Inuit societies in the Arctic that relied on fish and meat for millennia. In an experiment he conducted on himself in the late 1920s, Harvard anthropologist Vilhjalmur Stefansson spent an entire year eating only meat and suffered no ill effects according to doctors who monitored him. Ludwig does not contend that there is anything wrong with vegetables, fruits, and other unrefined carbs, he just makes the point that we *can* do without them. But on refined carbs, his message is clear: avoid them. After talking with Ludwig, I was never able to eat my usual rolled oats, white Italian bread, and white rice and beans with the same innocence—all of them are bad actors.

When I joined WW International, I noticed during our weekly meetings how often my fellow members talked about uncontrollable cravings for candy, ice cream, and non-diet soft drinks. In his 1972 book *Pure, White, and Deadly: How Sugar is Killing Us and What We Can Do to Stop It*, John Yudkin, a physician and professor at the University of London, presented a compelling argument that sugar is the worst nutrition offender of all. Among other ills, Yudkin believed that the ubiquitous sweetener is the primary cause of heart attacks. In doing so, he directly contradicted the findings of American researcher Ancel Keys, who had singled out saturated fat as Public Enemy Number-One in the epidemic of coronary disease.

Yudkin pulled no punches: "Avoid sugar, I say, and you are less likely to become fat, run into nutritional deficiency, have a heart attack, get diabetes or dental decay or a duodenal ulcer, and perhaps you also reduce your chances of getting gout, dermatitis, and some forms of cancer, and in general increase your lifespan." His work being questioned, Keys struck back viciously, claiming that Yudkin had little evidence for his position that sugar caused heart disease and that what evidence he had wouldn't withstand even the most basic criticism. Undeterred, Yudkin contended that his research showed that, while there was a moderate correlation between deaths from heart ailments and fat consumption, there was a far closer relationship between coronary disease and sugar intake. He insisted that he could make two statements that no one—not even Keys—could refute. "First, there is no biological need for sugar; all human nutritional needs can be met in full without having to take a single spoon of white or brown or raw sugar, on its own or in any food or drink," Yudkin maintained. Secondly, if only a small fraction of what is already known about the effects of sugar were to be revealed in relation to any other material used as a food additive, that material would be promptly banned." At the very least, he felt he had acquired enough evidence to make it worthwhile to thoroughly investigate sugar as a coronary villain.

In a key experiment, Yudkin carefully cataloged the typical food intake of a group of nineteen young men. After putting them all on a baseline diet, he had the subjects replace the starchy carbohydrates in their diets with the same number of calories of sugar, making as few other changes as possible. Over two weeks, blood triglycerides and cholesterol rose in all the participants, and one-third of them also packed on about five pounds. These changes almost entirely disappeared when the men returned to their original diets. Yudkin theorized that consuming sugar leads to weight gain in many people, and that weight gain in turn predisposes humans to heart disease.

"SUGAR IS NOT A FOOD. IT IS A FOOD ADDITIVE, AND IT IS A CHEMICAL TOXIN."

—DR. ROBERT LUSTIG

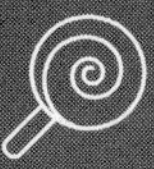
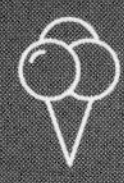
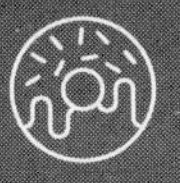
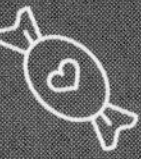

1. SUGAR GOES INTO THE BODY

2. THE BODY DIGESTS SUGAR QUICKLY, CAUSING A SURGE OF GLUCOSE IN THE BLOODSTREAM

3. GLUCOSE GOES TO THE LIVER, WHERE IT'S TURNED INTO FAT AND THE EXCESS IS EXPORTED TO FAT CELLS

4. THE PANCREAS RELEASES A SURGE OF INSULIN IN RESPONSE TO THE GLUCOSE

5. INSULIN RESISTS LEPTIN (THE HORMONE THAT TELLS THE BRAIN THE BODY IS SATED)

6. THE INSULIN CAUSES FAT TO INCREASE

Despite Yudkin's results, Keys triumphed. Yudkin's work was buried beneath the arguments that saturated fat was the true villain. Yudkin was all but forgotten by the scientific community.

When I was a child, a few stalks of sugarcane grew outside the kitchen window of my parents' cottage in Jamaica. The dull green, bamboolike plants with their white tassels soared above the building's eaves. With a few whacks from the fearsome machete, which accompanied him everywhere, the yardman severed the stalks into sections that I could transport in my back pocket. I used my penknife for the final stage of prep, whittling away the woody outer "rind" to expose the white interior and cutting off one generous mouthful at a time. My reward was a sweet treat, although accessing it required long, ruminative chewing, which would have won high praises from Horace Fletcher, the Great Masticator. Eventually, all that remained in my mouth was a tasteless wad of fiber. By permitting me to enjoy that sugarcane habit, my parents were not being negligent. For starters, cane in its just-harvested state is 13 to 18 percent sugar—about the same content as an apple. And all that time spent chewing meant that the sugar entered my digestive system slowly, so my blood glucose levels stayed fairly level.

The story of the consumption of sugar throughout the world would have been inconsequential, limited to a few populations in Southeast Asia, where the plant was domesticated, if someone in India around 500 CE had not figured out a way to circumvent all that tedious jaw grinding. Chopping and crushing the plants, pressing out the liquid, and refining it produces white, nearly pure crystals of sucrose, the chemical compound we commonly call sugar. Sucrose consists of two conjoined sugar molecules: glucose and fructose. Anyone who wants to lose weight—or anyone who eats, for that matter—should keep this simple chemical formula in mind. With only two molecules to deal with, the digestive system breaks down sugar much more rapidly than it processes more complex substances. According to food historian Sidney Mintz, author of *Sweetness and Power: The Place of Sugar in Modern History*, those glucose-fructose crystals remain the only chemical substance we consume in "practically pure form as a staple food."

Studies conducted in the mid-1900s showed that Americans satisfied their appetite for this chemical at the expense of the more complex, harder-to-digest carbohydrates found naturally in fruits, vegetables, and whole-grain breads. Between 1909 and the early 1970s, we reduced the percentage of these healthful carbs in our diet by nearly half, while the portion supplied by sugar shot up by more than half.

Things got a lot worse beginning in the 1970s with the widespread introduction of high-fructose corn syrup (HFCS), a product manufactured from cornstarch. It is "high" because it has slightly more fructose than regular corn syrup, but chemically it's almost identical to sucrose, being composed of glucose, some glucose that has been converted into fructose, and fructose. HFCS affects metabolism in ways similar to sugar, and tastes as sweet. But it has two big benefits—for food companies' profits, that is. One, corn, its raw source, is grown widely in this country (and heavily subsidized by our tax dollars); and two, HFCS is cheaper than sugar, which is derived from cane or beets. Beverage and food-processing companies began loading HFCS into nearly everything they produced. Fueled by the inexpensive sweetener, Americans' consumption of all sugars soared from less than 20 pounds a year in the early 1900s to about 150 pounds, and our rate of obesity rose more than fourfold.

Robert Lustig, a researcher at the University of California, San Francisco, and author of the 2013 bestseller *Fat Chance: Beating the Odds Against Sugar, Processed Food, Obesity, and Disease,* describes himself as a Yudkin disciple. As such, he is one of the leading advocates for cutting

SUGAR RUSH

SUGAR BEETS
SUGARCANE

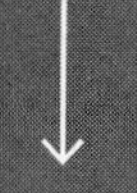

SUCROSE
50% GLUCOSE & 50% FRUCTOSE

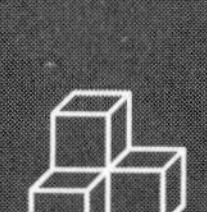

MORE THAN TWO DOZEN
FORMS OF SUGAR

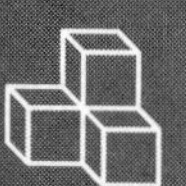

CORN

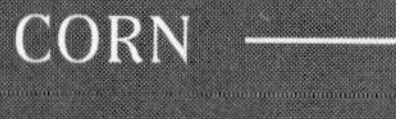

CORN SYRUP:
100% GLUCOSE

CORNSTARCH

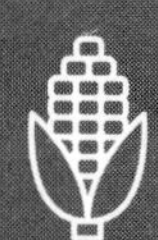

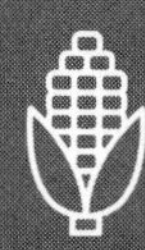

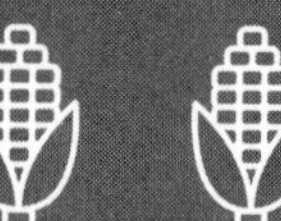

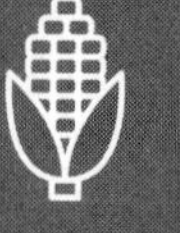

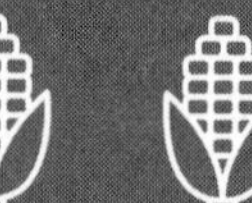

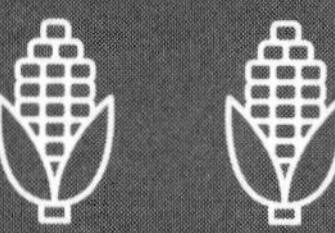

HIGH-FRUCTOSE CORN SYRUP:
GLUCOSE, GLUCOSE
CONVERTED INTO
FRUCTOSE, AND FRUCTOSE

FRUCTOSE:
7X MORE
DAMAGING

sugar consumption. "Every successful diet in history restricts sugar," he told me when I sought his advice on losing weight. "Sugar is not a food. It is a food additive, and it is a chemical toxin."

Working in the years prior to the 1970s, Yudkin did not have the information necessary to decipher the full spectrum of the health damage caused by excessive sugar consumption, nor did he discover exactly how the harm was done. I asked Lustig to explain how sugar would fatten me according to the most recent research. He said that it begins with how sugar affects insulin. Our body digests sugar rapidly, creating a surge of glucose in the blood. The pancreas releases insulin to deal with the glucose. "The more insulin, the more fat," Lustig said. "Anything that makes your body produce insulin will make you fat. Insulin makes fat. Period."

High insulin levels work another way against anyone who is trying to lose weight. They create resistance to a hormone called leptin. When all is well, fat cells secrete leptin, and the hormone informs the brain that the body has enough stored energy, causing you to feel full and satisfied. But if your body has been made resistant to leptin by too much insulin, you still feel hungry even after a big meal. You've eaten plenty, but your system reacts to what it perceives as a lack of nourishment by slowing down in an effort to conserve energy. You remain famished, which causes you to eat more, opening the way for even greater weight gain.

That's only half the sugar story, according to Lustig. "Remember, sugar and HFCS are made of two different molecules, one glucose, the other fructose," he said. "And fructose is seven times as bad for you as glucose." Unlike glucose, which goes into the bloodstream after being digested, fructose is sent to the liver to be metabolized. Confronted with too much fructose for it to handle, the liver turns the excess into fat, some of which is exported to the fat cells, which drives weight gain, some of which remains in the liver as fat, which drives higher insulin levels. "We're getting frucked," said Lustig.

One obvious way to make an end run around sugar and still enjoy soda, ice cream, and sweetened coffee would be to opt for zero- or low-calorie foods and drinks with artificial sweeteners, like saccharin, aspartame, and sucralose. Many studies confirm that zero-calorie beverages do, indeed, help you reduce, and several of my sweets-loving fellow Weight Watchers found them to be effective tools. Unfortunately, a conflicting body of research shows that fake sweeteners are no better for you—and may be worse in some cases—than the real thing. In a paper published in 2016, Susan Swithers, of Purdue University, examined dozens of studies that compared sugar-sweetened products to those using artificial sweeteners. She concluded that consumers of sugar substitutes may be at risk of excessive weight gain, heart disease, and type 2 diabetes. She noted that consumption of sugar-free soft drinks in the United States between 1960 and 2000 increased in tandem with the rates of overweight and obesity. The rates of metabolic syndrome (a condition associated with cardiovascular disease and diabetes) rose by as much as 100 percent among consumers of fake sugars.

M. Yanina Pepino, of the University of Illinois, administered sucralose, a calorie-free sweetener, to a group of obese men and women. She found that the sweetener drove up levels of glucose in the blood and triggered the release of fat-generating insulin by as much as 20 percent, and that the levels of insulin stayed higher for longer than they did in a group of control subjects.

Theories vary on why this happens, according to Swithers' review of the scientific literature. Sweet tastes may weaken the feeling of satiety, leading to the consumption of more food than normal. Experiments conducted by a group of Australian researchers suggest that when the body tastes something it perceives as sweet, it readies itself for the blast of calories that real sugars normally provide. When those calories fail to arrive on cue, as happens when you consume sugar substitutes, the brain thinks it is being starved and urges the body to eat calorie-dense food.

Today, the average American gulps the equivalent of nearly twenty teaspoons of sugar a day—more than twice the amount recommended by the American Heart Association. Of course, no one sprinkles twenty teaspoons of sugar on their breakfast cereal or scoops that much Into their coffee and tea. Food processors add the rest, and not just in the obvious foods, like cookies, ice cream treats, breakfast cereals, and candy bars. When I examined some random labels during a trip to the supermarket, I found that prepared spaghetti sauce, frozen battered fish fillets, most bread, salad dressing, and crackers were minefields for anyone wanting to avoid sugar. Knowing that sugar has become a dirty word for some nutrition-conscious consumers, the food industry ties itself in linguistic knots to avoid using the dreaded *S* word. Lustig told me to beware of the following terms on food packaging:

Agave nectar
Barley malt
Brown rice syrup
Caramel
Carob syrup
Corn syrup
Crystalline fructose
Dextran
Dextrose
Ethyl maltol
Florida crystals
Galactose

THE AMERICAN SUGAR RUSH

OUTCOME

OBESITY RATES HAVE QUADRUPLED

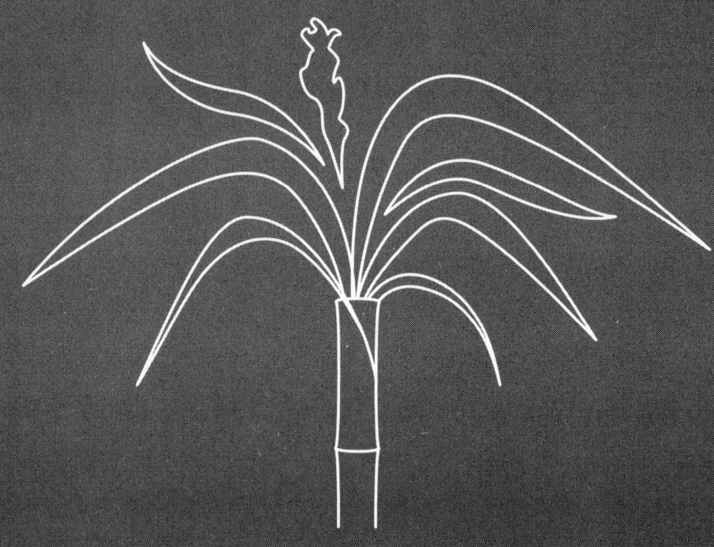

EARLY 1900S

AMERICANS CONSUMED LESS THAN
20 POUNDS OF SUGAR ANNUALLY

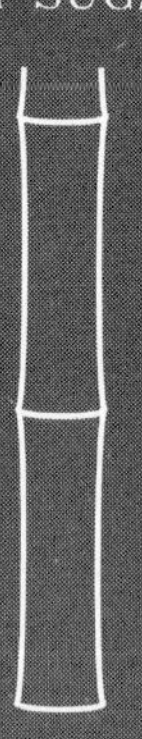

TODAY

AMERICANS CONSUME ABOUT
150 POUNDS OF SUGAR EACH YEAR

Glucose
Golden syrup
Lactose
Maltose
Malt syrup
Refiner's syrup
Rice syrup

They are sugar by another name, every one. The very presence of a label listing ingredients and a nutritional profile on a food container should be a red flag, according to Lustig. "A food label is a warning label," he said, adding that the words *fat-free* are also a good indication that high levels of sugar have been added to a product to make up for the lack of fat.

Fortunately, Lustig advised me, there is one way to counteract fructose's toxic effects. Eat fiber. In nature, the sweetener is never found in its pure state. It's usually in fiber-rich fruits and vegetables. "When God made the poison, he also packaged it with the antidote," Lustig said. "Fiber slows digestion and absorption." This gives you time to fully metabolize what you eat. Also, because fiber is bulky, you fill up quickly, automatically consuming fewer calories. And, as my boyhood sugarcane consumption showed, fibrous foods must be chewed longer than those lacking fiber, which gives the body even more time to receive its satiety signal. "There is only one good way to get fiber," said Lustig. "From the source. Eat real food that came out of the ground or food from an animal that ate real food that came out of the ground."

As Yudkin asserted, "Many people lose excessive weight very successfully by giving up sugar, or by severely restricting it."

Unfortunately for me, though, I'm not many people. I'm blessed with whatever you'd call the opposite of a sweet tooth. I rarely eat packaged foods. I almost never have dessert (though I've been known to purloin a spoonful or two of whatever my wife orders at restaurants). My coffee is black. I don't drink soft drinks of any kind. My only sugary shortcoming was the tablespoon of home-produced maple syrup I drizzled on top of my morning bowl of yogurt. And given the amount of exercise I get cutting and splitting firewood and lugging buckets of maple sap through knee-deep snow to our sugar house where I boil it down into syrup, I think even Yudkin would give me a pass on that. I had to search elsewhere for my bad actors.

I once regarded alcohol as a buddy. It gave instant relief from stress, enhanced my meals, and made me more outgoing. I dreaded the thought of any social gathering, particularly one where I would encounter strangers, without a drink in hand. Alcohol had been a big part of my life for more than fifty years. My mother and father were typical 1950s upper-middle-class suburban drinkers. Today we'd call them alcoholics. At our house, not a day passed without the sacred ritual of cocktail hour being observed, and the weekends and vacations were a series of extended parties with their friends, all drinkers. Both my mother and brother eventually did time in rehab to treat their alcohol issues.

I had gone to a leading university that had a well-earned reputation for being a bastion of hard study and harder play, which meant beer, beer, and more beer. After college, I got a job at a newspaper. In the waning days of the swashbuckling reporter, a deadline rarely passed without the newsroom emptying as we merrily paraded across the street to the nearest bar. Of course, I wasn't entirely ignorant about the caloric content of booze. But I knew lots of people—coworkers, friends, my parents—who drank at least as much as I did, and they were not obese. I had no idea, though, of just how awash in calories the stuff is. Per gram, alcohol packs more calories than carbohydrates or protein and is second only to fat. When I dropped into our town's brew pub to quaff a single pint of craft-brewed IPA, I guzzled 300 calories—as many as there are in a generous slice of pepperoni pizza. At 125 calories each, the two glasses of red wine that I regularly enjoyed with dinner added 250 calories. The occasional martinis my wife and I sipped on the patio as the sun set on summer evenings delivered 180. And those are just estimates. As I learned from the WW app, I really had no idea how many calories I was getting or exactly how many drinks I consumed. How much, precisely, was the bartender drawing from the tap? At home, I never bothered to measure the wine that gurgled out of the bottle, or use a shot glass when mixing a drink. There is a reason they coined the term *home pour*. And that's not to mention all of those times that I dropped in for a single drink and succumbed to my buddies' entreaties to have just one more.

Many of us tell little white lies, even to ourselves, perhaps especially to ourselves, about how many drinks we have over the course of a day or week. Physicians know this. Doctor Dennis slipped me some inside info when he said that in medical school, he and his classmates were actually taught to add 50 percent to the number of drinks patients confess to consuming to arrive at an accurate figure of their booze intake. I hadn't factored that into my calculations.

Large though it may be, that high calorie content is only one of the dastardly set of tactics drinking was deploying to keep me fat—more than I had ever imagined. Studies suggest that I imbibed those boozy calories in addition to, not instead of, the number of food calories I ate on days when I didn't touch a drop. In an article published in The *American Journal of Clinical Nutrition*, Rosalind Breslow, of the National Institute on Alcohol Abuse and Alcoholism, and her associates reported that men who were mostly moderate drinkers consumed at least 400 calories more (the equivalent of a McDonald's Quarter Pounder) on days when they drank than on days when they abstained. The alcohol contributed about 265 of those calories.

I was always a glutton for the calorie-rich appetizers on offer at cocktail receptions. I blamed nervousness and weakened willpower after a drink or two. But it turns out that lack of self-discipline was not my problem. As they say, booze made me do it. British scientists found that, regardless of how much their research subjects had eaten, alcohol stimulated the same brain cells that are activated by starvation. This caused hunger pangs I normally would have experienced after a long period of not eating a thing. Although their experiments were conducted on mice, the researchers concluded that the phenomenon occurs across mammals.

We all know that excessive drinking can wreak havoc on the liver. It causes cirrhosis, of course. Fortunately, Doctor Dennis's tests showed I had no signs of that (which may say more about the hardiness of my liver than my drinking habits). But it can also lead to a condition called fatty liver, which is just what it sounds like: fat is stored in the liver, which adds pounds to your body and puts strain on the organ. As pleasant as I found the little buzz I got unwinding with a drink after a day's work, alcohol is essentially a neurotoxin—a poison. One of the many functions of the liver is to remove poisons from your blood. Ever diligent, the organ recognized the alcohol in my glass of wine for what it was and prioritized getting rid of it as quickly as possible. Yet it did so at the expense of processing calories from the other nutrients I was ingesting, causing them to be rerouted to fat cells instead of being used for energy. I experienced the same effect as a group of California men who in an experiment saw their metabolisms plummet by as much as 73 percent while their livers focused on getting rid of the alcohol in a couple of modest-size drinks.

One benefit I got from liquor, or so I thought, was a good night's sleep. After I'd had a few, I fell promptly into a deep, dreamless slumber. Alas,

Dr. Christopher Winter, of Charlottesville Neurology and Sleep Medicine, in Virginia, informed me that while alcohol may be a great sedative for helping you go to sleep, it is also one of the very best ways to ruin the rest of your night's sleep. "Alcohol suppresses deep sleep," he said. "And deep sleep is what makes us feel rested and refreshed."

Not being well rested can cause weight gain in several ways, according to Winter. First, when you are tired, you are less inclined to exercise—I know I am. But sleep deprivation can also lower your aversion to unhealthy foods and behaviors without your realizing it. Even at times when I had consumed too many drinks, I was still self-aware enough to toss the car keys to my wife. Yet in the sober light of the next morning, I'd often pick up a quick snack at a convenience store. I'd never associated that with the previous night's revelries, but Winter told me that even though I felt clearheaded, my judgment could still have been impaired, just enough to allow me to succumb to a temptation I would have made myself resist if I knew that booze was influencing my behavior.

A bad night's sleep also alters the rate at which your body metabolizes foods in as yet unexplained ways. The parts of the brain that tell us to eat are particularly active after a night of poor sleep. "That can lead to people to eat, not out of hunger, but out of fatigue," said Winter. A University of Chicago study showed that a group of young men had nearly 20 percent lower levels of leptin, a hormone that suppresses appetite, on mornings after they had been deprived of sleep. At the same time, they had about 30 percent higher levels ghrelin, a hormone that intensifies appetite. They experienced increased cravings for calorie-dense and high-carb foods. Other research shows that men ate between 385 and 560 calories more on days when they were sleep deprived than when they were well rested. It's paradoxical, but true. Sleeping, that most sedentary of human behaviors, can help us lose weight.

But what about the French Paradox and all those studies on the Mediterranean diet showing that alcohol, particularly red wine, is healthful? If I abstained in order to lose weight, was I missing out on the good that a drink can do? The Mayo Clinic says that moderate intake can, indeed, reduce your chances of dying from heart disease, stroke, and maybe even diabetes. But, the Mayo warns, the operative word here is *moderate*. I would describe their recommendations as extremely moderate. For women, the limit is one drink a day; men can have two. The reason for the difference? Men have higher levels of alcohol dehydrogenase, a liver enzyme that breaks down alcohol. If you exceed those limits, booze goes from being mildly beneficial to an outright scourge. Not only do you gain weight but your risk of cancer of the breast, mouth, throat, esophagus, and liver increases, as do the chances of having heart failure, stroke, and sudden death for those who already have heart disease—and that's just a short list. When I asked my cardiologist about the benefits of red wine, he said they were not so great that he would ever suggest someone take up drinking wine for heart health.

For a drinker like me who was trying to lose weight, there is a silver lining. Strong scientific evidence suggests that cutting back on alcohol can have profound effects. In the famous Framingham Heart Study, scientists who monitored participants observed that those who increased their alcohol consumption gained weight, but those who simply quit and changed nothing else experienced a mean weight loss of "several kilograms."

If having my fat melt away by the kilogram is not reason enough to raise a celebratory glass, I don't know what would be. A glass of sparkling water, that is.

CHAPTER TWELVE

BIG WINNERS

We all know the grim statistic: somewhere around 90-plus percent of dieters gain back all the weight they lose and sometimes put on more. But there are way more dieters than I ever imagined who have beaten those formidable odds. They number in the thousands. I learned about them when I went to Providence, Rhode Island, to meet with J. Graham Thomas, a psychologist who works in the field of behavioral medicine at the Warren Alpert Medical School of Brown University.

Thomas is a tall, soft-spoken, friendly man who sports a close-cropped beard and whose hair is just beginning to gray. He works out of an office that is noteworthy for its blandness and lack of the usual work-space photographs and tchotchkes. Like many nutrition experts I encountered, he is tall and borderline skinny. Although he treats participants in the hospital's weight-loss programs, a big part of Thomas's work involves studying members of a group with the Orwellian name National Weight Control Registry. Don't worry; it's not some secret government scheme to march us all onto scales and report the results to a central bureaucracy. Members sign up voluntarily. It's a tough club to join, and I would be delighted if someday I qualified for membership. To gain admittance, you have to have lost at least thirty pounds and kept them off for one year, although the average member has dropped sixty-six pounds and maintained that loss for five and a half years. A few have dropped as much as three hundred pounds.

The registry was founded in 1993 with the goal of determining if it was even possible to lose weight for the long term. At the time, most nutrition experts would have answered no. They were wrong. Since its inception, about twelve thousand people have joined the registry. The Brown researchers more than proved their original hypothesis: It may be hard, it may be rare, but a large group of Americans had done what I thought was, for me, impossible. Having shown that lasting weight loss was indeed a possibility, Thomas and his associates shifted the focus of the project and began to comb through data gleaned from member surveys to see how they'd done it. Maybe these weight-loss "champions" knew things that I and others could use to achieve similar long-term success.

In her book *Thin for Life: 10 Keys to Success from People Who Have Lost Weight and Kept It Off* (published in 1994 by Chapters, where I worked), Anne M. Fletcher interviewed a much smaller group, 160 people who

WHEN YOU LOSE WEIGHT,
YOUR METABOLISM *SLOWS*.

EXERCISE DOES THREE THINGS:

INCREASES METABOLISM

CONTROLS APPETITE

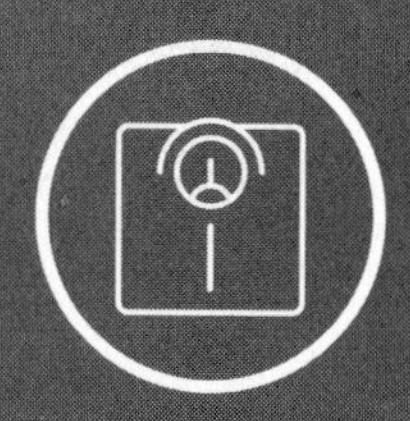

BURNS CALORIES

EXERCISE IS IMPORTANT FOR
MAINTAINING WEIGHT LOSS.

she called "masters." They had dropped at least twenty pounds and maintained their weight at the reduced level for at least three years. Like Thomas, she wanted to find their secrets. "Who better to tell you how to lose weight permanently than the very people who have done it," Fletcher wrote.

Both Thomas' and Fletcher's work reveal that the secret to weight loss is there is no single secret. "The more I looked at their answers to the question, 'When you were finally successful, how did you do it?' the more I was struck by the diversity of their answers. . . . *Their message—loud and clear—is that if you want to lose weight, you have to find what's best for you,*" Fletcher wrote.

Similarly, Thomas told me that members of the registry used a variety of methods to reach their goals. About half took the Frank Sinatra approach—doing it their way. The other half did it with the help of a program. Some lost weight in a flash, while others did so at a glacial pace, taking as long as fourteen years. "But the key," said Thomas, "is to avoid extreme anything. Members who go to extremes tend to relapse. It's not the eating plan you follow that's important, it's how well you follow it. We encourage people to do whatever they can stick with. One thing that can derail you is feeling deprived, so keep eating the things you enjoy, but try to modify your intake. That's a lot easier than completely giving up a food or category of food. Most members don't lose on their first or even second attempts. They try several different approaches. There is considerable variability."

Some members of the registry, the fortunate ones, have little trouble finding their demons and dealing with them. "In our clinical studies, we've had men lose fifty pounds by switching from regular beer to light. If you're drinking a lot of beer, small changes like that can make a big difference. We've seen the same thing with fast food. Cutting back on visits to your favorite chain restaurant can have a huge effect," Thomas said. "But other people have lost weight by making little changes across the board."

Long-term losers employ another simple, highly effective trick. The vast majority weigh themselves, usually at least once a week. And the ones who weigh in the most frequently were significantly less likely to put on pounds than those who avoided the scale. "It's much easier to correct a five-pound bump than one of twenty pounds," he said. "You catch the problem earlier by weighing in. I mean, you wouldn't drive a car without a speedometer. You can also monitor food intake, fat grams, calories—whatever you want. The important thing it to keep track and have some sort of metric."

Critically, when it comes to health benefits, a little weight loss goes a long way. Thomas says his research subjects start seeing clinically important improvements in their sense of well-being after dropping as little as 3 percent of their weight. Those improvements become significant at 5 percent, even among those who remain technically obese. "It's better to lose a modest amount of weight and keep it off for a long time than it is to lose a huge amount and gain it back," Thomas said.

Although almost all registry members initially lost their weight by changing their diets, they keep it off by exercising—a lot. They average an hour per day, and burn off between 2,250 and 2,600 calories through exercise per week, equal to a little more than a day's recommended intake for a man of my size. But again, they are a highly variable group. About one-quarter burn fewer than 1,000 calories exercising, a third burn more than 3,000. And the workouts need not be hard. Simply walking is the most common activity.

"When you lose weight, you lose by changing your diet," Thomas said. "If you only change your physical activity, that alone won't make you lose much weight. But while exercise might not be an important thing for weight loss, it is one of the most important things for *maintaining* it. When you lose weight, your metabolism slows. If you take two people who both weigh 150 pounds, and one always weighed that amount and the other had to lose 50 pounds to get there, then the one who lost the weight will have a lower metabolism, and it will stay low. Exercising raises your metabolism." Exercise has a twofold effect. You not only get the benefit of the extra calories you burn while exercising, but your metabolism stays higher throughout the day—like a bonus. And exercise also helps you control your appetite, although Thomas says scientists have not discovered how it works.

The registry's members employed some tactics I knew would not work for me. The majority, but by no means all, lost their weight on lower-fat regimes. I had trouble sticking to a program like that during my stint as a Dean Ornish follower. Very few participants drink sugar-sweetened beverages regularly, but a little over half do consume artificially sweetened drinks. I consume neither, although like the champions, I do imbibe lots of water. A large number also limited their diets to relatively few foods, which they ate consistently. "It's something we psychologists call sensory specific satiety," Thomas said. "If you eat the same things all the time, you tend to eat less of them. People in the program eat the same thing over and over, and that protects them from the wide variety of tempting food out there. Access to that variety promotes weight gain." Sorry, Professor Thomas, to me variety is the spice of life—literally. I'd call it sensory deprivation.

Regardless of how they originally dropped the extra pounds, registry members continue to work on weight loss all the time. This, however, does not condemn them to a life of sustaining superhuman discipline and fretting over everything they eat. According Thomas, it not only gets easier to keep off unwanted pounds as time passes, the pleasures from being in better physical shape and enjoying a healthful diet can eventually eclipse the effort expended. Over time, they find they no longer rely on as many strategies to keep off the weight.

For me, the visit to Thomas was good news. It was possible that I could begin a virtuous cycle—the more I lost, the easier it would become to keep it off. And if Thomas was right, that would hold true regardless of what path (or paths) I'd take to get there.

CHAPTER THIRTEEN

MINI ME

Nearly four years have passed since that game-changing appointment, when I sat on the examining table while Doctor Dennis showed me the grim numbers on his laptop.

As a dieter, I flunked.

But here's the catch: That day in Doctor Dennis's office, I weighed 238 pounds. I'm down to 212 today. That's 26 pounds to the good. For the first time in three decades, I have dropped out of the ranks of the four in ten Americans who are clinically obese. Given the physiques of all the men in my family, I doubt I'll ever be svelte, unless they repeal Mendel's laws of inheritance. But I am now able to bicycle, hike, and cross-country ski without gasping for air. Shirts and pants fit better. I've even had to bore new holes in some of my belts so that they effectively keep my trousers aloft.

But the real changes are unseen. My blood pressure has dropped from a way-too-high 164 over 86—and that was controlled by swallowing a 300mg irbesartan tablet (the maximum dose allowed) every morning. Now my blood pressure is 112 over 62, comfortably within the ideal range, and Doctor Dennis has taken me off blood-pressure meds for the first time since the late 1990s. My cholesterol levels have tumbled from unhealthy heights to normal.

What gives?

For starters, I now know why diets fail so consistently, at least for me, and I suspect for a large number of dieters. I will never go on one again. Diets are based on the premise that their authors have found a new, better way to eat and they try to convince you to consume food in a way that fits with their strictures. To succeed, you must force yourself to adhere to their rules. That's attacking the weight problem from the precisely wrong direction. You should lead a diet, not follow one. What you eat and how you do so are deeply personal activities, right up there with sex. They are nobody else's damn business, and I, like most, resent someone telling me how I should tend to such matters, no matter how well-meaning the advice. For me, successful weight loss began when I examined what I ate and how I ate it, then started making changes—just tinkering around the edges at first—to see what took off pounds and what kept them in place.

Uncontrollable cravings never caused me to fall off a diet. Mostly the cause was sheer boredom, working in tandem with frustration. I learned early on that following recipes in diet books doomed me to failure. Too many of them are poorly edited, untested, and simply do not work. It's not enough to reduce the fat or sugar in a dish, which seems to be a common tactic of diet-recipe developers. I know this from personal experience, having once edited a food magazine that emphasized healthful, low-fat recipes. For weeks, our test kitchen tried to come up with a better version of good-ol' American apple pie. Called in to taste one final, stripped-down version, the staff dietitian grimaced and pleaded, "Can't we just tell readers to take smaller slices?" A wise woman.

Recipes produced under the supervision of nutritionists, doctors, and scientists lack the depth of culinary knowledge and soul that is the hallmark of any worthwhile cookbook. But my biggest complaint was that none of them fit with the way my wife and I actually cook and eat. Sorry, I don't have time to chop for a half hour before lunch. I don't want to separate egg yolks from the whites before making an omelet. I distrust every food labeled with the prefix *low-*, as in low-fat, low-salt, or low-anything. The same applies to the suffix *free*. I'd sooner do without pasta than opt for the whole-wheat kind. And don't get me started on gluten-free stand-ins for bread. As if diet books' individual recipes were not bad enough, I could never stick to their three-meals-a-day, weeks-long, set-in-stone menu plans. I could tolerate such ordeals for maybe five days, then I lapsed, usually with a mighty sigh of relief.

Interestingly, most early diet books were brief and without recipes. William Banting's wildly influential *Letter on Corpulence Addressed to the Public*, written in 1863, had no recipes and was only 11 pages long—including addenda and appendices. Diet book inflation has been afflicting us ever since. Horace Fletcher's *Fletcherism* came out in 1913 at 86 pages. Five years later, Lulu Hunt Peters's *Diet and Health with Key to the Calories*, the first modern diet bestseller, had 109 pages. Dallas Hartwig and Melissa Urban's *The Whole30*, by contrast, is 432 pages long, more than 200 of which are taken up by recipes. And it's far from the fattest of the modern crop of diet books. Something in me suspects the publishers are responsible for such overstuffed tomes. Throw in a hundred or so recipes as an afterthought, and bookstore customers will think they're getting a better deal. No wonder dieters give up.

When we met, Arthur Agatston, whose South Beach books are themselves thick with recipes, admitted that people who master the science behind his diet and then incorporate that into their meals are more likely to succeed than those who rely on following his recipes to the letter. Once I began doing that, I found it easier to stick within the parameters of whatever program I endured at the time. My version of ratatouille is a lot easier to make than Dean Ornish's, is tastier, and still falls within his stringent low-fat limits. The same is true of my meatless chili.

Dutifully following formal diets and programs did teach me some valuable lessons. Although I dropped out of Weight Watchers after a couple of months, the point-tracking app that came with my membership made it abundantly clear that I would never lose weight unless I cut way back on how much cheese I snacked on. I had never thought that my habit was enough to materially enlarge my waistline. But day after day, those little nibbles made me blow past my Weight Watchers' points limit. Now, like Pépin, I treat myself to much smaller amounts of tastier cheese less often. The point is that there are useful weight-loss tips between the covers of diet books, enough that it might not be a bad idea to pick up a few to see if anything inside fits with your eating patterns. And who knows, you might be one of the lucky dieters who manage to lose weight and keep it off by adhering to a specific regime. Congratulations, if you are.

But I learned far more from the cultures that remain healthy and avoid excess weight just by going about the business of eating as they traditionally have. Importantly, I have adjusted their approaches to fit my own tastes and lifestyle. In the process, I have radically changed my diet—one step at a time.

The physically active, teetotaler, near-vegetarian Seventh-day Adventists prompted me to rethink my consumption of alcohol and meat and to incorporate exercise into my daily routine, as did the findings of the National Weight Control Registry. I tried joining a gym, but didn't enjoy workouts there. I love to walk and cycle, however, and weather permitting, I get in at least an hour a day. At first it required some self-discipline, but now I feel bad if a day goes by without my exercising. I even bought a standing desk, mindful of the warning from the feisty leader of that Loma Linda aerobics class that "sitting is the enemy." I also eat a handful of nuts with my breakfast because I find they help keep me comfortably full until lunchtime. And if the results of the Adventist studies are correct, I may be doing my heart a big favor, too.

In Greece, I discovered that I could easily make thoroughly satisfying main courses out of vegetables, especially during the summer months, when our garden and local farmers' markets overflow with fresh produce, provided that I liberally poured on olive oil. Stints as a vegetarian taught me that meat will always play a part in my diet, just not nearly as large a part as it once did. Its place of prominence has been usurped by beans of all types, despite the warnings of The Whole30 diet that beans can be bad for you. With apologies to Jerry Seinfeld (who traded a suit for a meal and then couldn't close out the trade when the other guy kept ordering soup and claiming that didn't count as a meal), I've also learned that soup can, indeed, be a meal. A glorious, satisfying one. Now we enjoy spicy white bean stew with broccoli rabe, red lentil soup, mushroom barley soup, Cuban black bean soup, and meatless chili. I now no longer have eggs every morning, opting for zero-percent-fat yogurt most days. I eat very little of what I call "boy food," a hunk of grilled meat, a starch, and a veg. Now it's a smaller piece of lean meat and a couple of vegetables, or very often three or four vegetables and no meat.

The so-called French Paradox turns out to be no paradox after all. I emulate Pépin by avoiding between-meal snacks. If I succumb, an apple, pear, or tangerine usually tides me over. I rarely eat lunch at my desk, instead I leave the outbuilding on our property that houses my office and walk to the house for a tuna salad with vegetables chopped into it or leftovers from a previous dinner. Sandwiches have vanished. My wife and I have always sat down each night we're home together and enjoyed a proper dinner. But now I'm taking somewhat smaller portions than previously, especially of foods high in fat and calories. I still have a way to go, but I am getting better at not heading back to the stove for second helpings.

And no matter what we have, we make it a point to eat the highest quality we can find—the freshest fruits and vegetables, when they are at their seasonal prime; wild fish; and grass-fed beef or pastured pork (rarely). Yeah, foods like these cost more, but they taste better, and I find that I am easily satisfied consuming less than I do when confronted with lower-quality fare. The French taught me that one of the most important ingredients in any successful diet is joy, and my new way of eating delivers way more of that than my previous diet.

But the most important lesson I learned from cultures with a less dysfunctional relationship with food than ours came from Mireille Guiliano, who recommended identifying and dealing with what she called usual suspects in *French Women Don't Get Fat*. I ruthlessly cut back (or eliminated) the bad actors that once made their way into my stomach. I zeroed in on the refined carbs in my diet. Out went white bread. When I found that my home-baked whole-wheat bread caused me to put on weight because it was so good that I ate way too much, that also went by the wayside. Our expensive toaster now serves as a stand on which we keep the kitchen radio. Brown rice stands in for white. Pasta of any sort has become rarer. I'm embarrassed to admit that I love potato chips. I often succumbed to my weakness by mindlessly stopping in at gas stations and leaving with a bottle of water and a bag of Lays, with its forty grams of processed carbs and 410 calories—more than I typically consume at breakfast or lunch. It seemed like a tiny sin at the time, but by kicking that one habit, I saved more than 2,000 calories a week. Eliminating these and other ultraprocessed carbohydrates required minimal sacrifice. Standing on the bathroom scale a few times a week (another new, painless habit) showed these steps helped me begin losing.

Alcohol was another story. A friend of mine once lost weight by limiting himself to two glasses of wine a day. I tried to kid myself by thinking I could emulate him. I could not. Finally, I had to admit that I'm one of those people who find it much easier to resist taking my first drink of the day than my second or third, by which time much of my self-restraint has drained away. Ultimately, I decided that I needed to abandon booze entirely. I won't lie and say it was easy. Just necessary. I started attending group sessions at a nearby medical center and managed to kick the habit. During a gathering early on, when I said that my goal was to lose weight for health reasons, the woman sitting next to me confided, "The pounds will fall off *sooo* fast."

And they did.

I remain very much a work in progress. For one thing, I still can't keep up with my wife on ski trails. More weight needs to be lost. But if I'm not mistaken, I saw the faintest hint of a smile on Doctor Dennis's face when he looked at his computer screen during a recent checkup.

BARRY'S PERSONAL REGIMEN

JOY OVER COMFORT

DO THIS

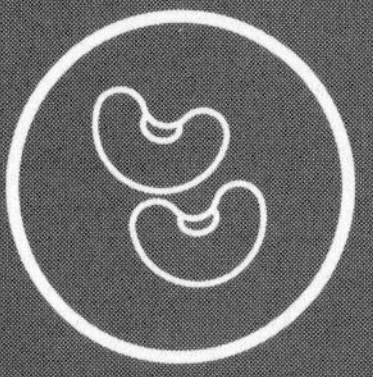

MORE BEANS

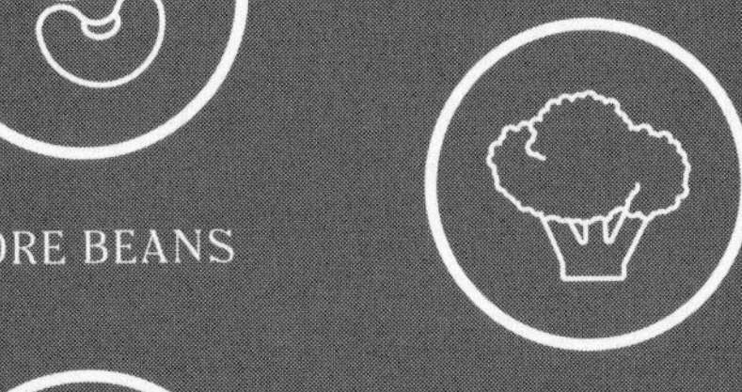

MORE VEGETABLES

FAT FROM OLIVE OIL

CYCLE OR WALK
ONE HOUR PER DAY

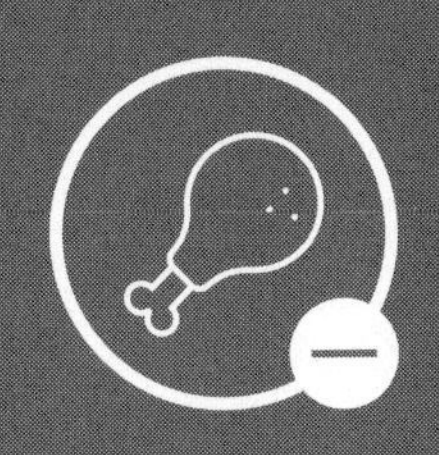

LESS MEAT

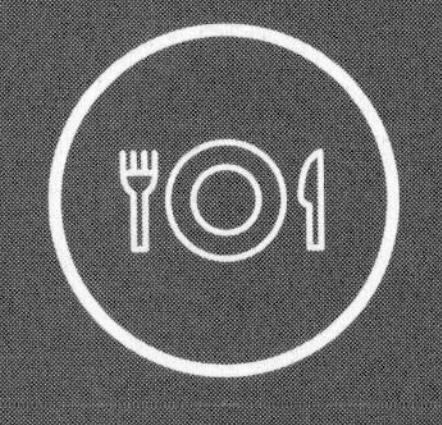

SMALLER AMOUNTS
OF HIGHER QUALITY
INGREDIENTS

NOT THIS

NO SNACKING

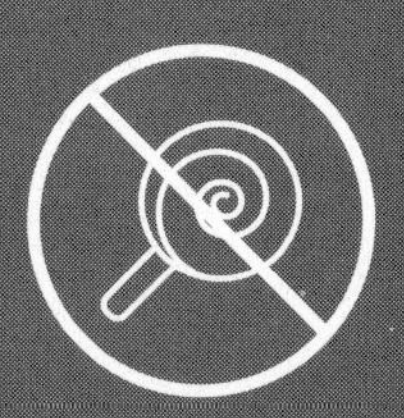

NO SUGAR

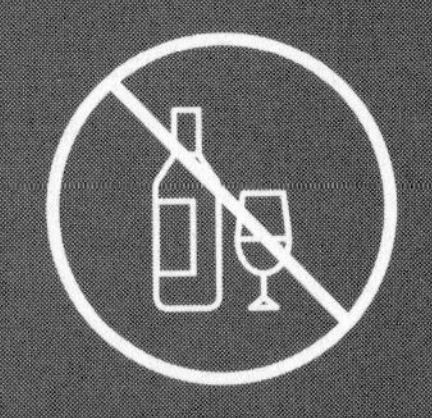

NO BOOZE

NO SANDWICHES

Precursors to Late-Twentieth-Century Diets

1830s—SYLVESTER GRAHAM

No: meat, coffee, tea, salt, pepper, spices, sauces, mustard, yeast

Yes: vegetables, fruit, nuts, water

1863—ELLEN G. WHITE

No: meat, alcohol, spices, sauces, coffee, tea

Yes: vegetables, fruit, whole grains

1864—WILLIAM BANTING

Publishes *Letter on Corpulence Addressed to the Public*

1865—ELLEN G. WHITE

Forms the Western Health Reform Institute in Battle Creek, Michigan

1874—JOHN HARVEY KELLOGG

Joins the Western Health Reform Institute;

prescribes diet of grapes, exclusively, for high blood pressure

1880s—JAMES HENRY SALISBURY

Promotes his Salisbury System of Weight Reduction

No: vegetables, starches

Yes: 3 pounds rump steak, 1 pound codfish, 3 quarts hot water

1887—WILLIAM OLIN ATWATER

Introduces concept of calories as unit of measure

EARLY 1900s—JAMES RAYMOND DEVEREUX
Recommends meatless diet in three meals:
Meal one—only vegetables
Meal two—only fruit
Meal three—only nuts

1913—HORACE FLETCHER
Introduces diet regimen of chewing food until liquified, spitting out remaining solids

1920—CABBAGE SOUP DIET
Only cabbage soup

1920s—HOLLYWOOD DIET (GRAPEFRUIT DIET)
Grapefruit, melba toast, straight coffee, celery, lettuce, tomato, an occasional egg

1929—DR. WILLIAM HAY
Warns against consuming protein and carbohydrates simultaneously

1934—GEORGE HARROP
700 to 1,000 calories per day from bananas, skim milk, and minimal roughage

1964—ROBERT CAMERON
Publishes *The Drinking Man's Diet;*
limit carbohydrates, but enjoy two martinis with a steak in béarnaise sauce

NOTES

Chapter One: Forty Unwanted Pounds

Page 3 **Joining the two-thirds:** See Lin Yang and Graham A. Colditz, "Prevalence of Overweight and Obesity in the United States, 2007–2012," *JAMA Internal Medicine* 175 no. 8 (August 2015): 1412–13, jamanetwork.com/journals/jamainternalmedicine/fullarticle/2323411.

Page 3 **I chose a regimen called The Whole30:** See Melissa Urban and Dallas Hartwig, *The Whole30: The 30-Day Guide to Total Health and Food Freedom* (Boston: Houghton Mifflin Harcourt, 2015).

Page 7 **another variation on the paleo diets:** See S. Boyd Eaton, Melvin Konner, "Paleolithic Nutrition—A Consideration of Its Nature and Current Implications," *New England Journal of Medicine* 312 (January 31, 1985): 283–89, www.ncbi.nlm.nih.gov/pubmed/2981409.

Page 8 **The paleo response:** See Michael Pollan, *In Defense of Food: An Eater's Manifesto* (New York: Penguin Press, 2008), 148.

Page 10 **constitutes a healthful diet:** See U. S. Department of Health and Human Services and U. S. Department of Agriculture, *2015–2020 Dietary Guidelines for Americans*, 8th edition, 2015, www.dietaryguidelines.gov/current-dietary-guidelines/2015-2020-dietary-guidelines.

Page 11 **In an interview:** See David Brooks, "Nashua Native Taking Nutrition Program on National Tour," *Nashua Telegraph*, May 16, 2015, www.nashuatelegraph.com/life/health-lifestyle/2015/05/16/nashua-native-taking-nutrition-program-on-national-tour. See also Melissa Urban's post on the Whole30 Blog, February 8, 2012.

Page 11 **According to a survey of nutrition experts:** See "U. S. News Best 35 Diets Overall," *U. S. News & World Report*, January 2, 2020, health.usnews.com/best-diet/best-diets-overall.

Page 12 **A paper by Yaguang Zheng:** See Yaguang Zheng et al., "Patterns of Self-Weighing Behavior and Weight Change in a Weight Loss Trial," *International Journal of Obesity* 40, no. 9 (September 2016): 1392–96, www.ncbi.nlm.nih.gov/pubmed/27113642.

Page 12 **According to the CDC:** See U. S. Department of Health and Human Services Centers for Disease Control and Prevention, "Keeping a Lapse from Becoming a Relapse," *Lifestyle Coach Facilitation Guide: Post Core*: 5, www.cdc.gov/diabetes/prevention/pdf/postcurriculum_session11.pdf.

Page 12 **According to Marketdata Enterprises:** for earnings of weight management industry, see John LaRosa, "Top 9 Things to Know about the Weight Loss Industry," Market Research Blog, March 6, 2019, blog.marketresearch.com/u.s.-weight-loss-industry-grows-to-72-billion. For value of produce, see "Retail Sales of Produce in the United States in 2018, by Type," Statista, www.statista.com/statistics/537716/us-dollar-sales-produce. For diet and fitness book sales, see Regina Nuzzo, "Diet Hooks," *Los Angeles Times*, March 10, 2008.

Page 13 **In a 2007 *American Psychologist* article:** See Traci Mann et al., "Medicare's Search for Effective Obesity Treatments: Diets are Not the Answer," *American Psychologist* 62, no. 3 (April 2007): 220–33, psycnet.apa .org/record/2007-04834-008.

Page 13 **In 1959, researchers conducted:** See Albert Stunkard and Mavis McLaren Hume, "The Results of Treatment for Obesity: Review of the Literature and Report of a Series," *Archives of Internal Medicine* 103, no.1 (January 1959): 79–85, jamanetwork.com/journals/jamainternalmedicine/ article-abstract/562795.

Page 13 **"We've spent decades counting calories":** See David Ludwig, *Always Hungry? Conquer Cravings, Retrain Your Fat Cells, and Lose Weight Permanently* (New York: Grand Central, 2016), 28.

Chapter Two: Instant Results

Page 16 **I chose a program called The Master Cleanse:** See Stanley A. Burroughs, *The Master Cleanser* (Riverside, CA: Burroughs Books, 1976).

Page 16 **celebrities such as Beyoncé Knowles:** See Lola Ogunnaike, "I Heard It Through the Diet Grapevine," *The New York Times,* December 19, 2016, www.nytimes .com/2006/12/10/fashion/10cleanse.html.

Page 16 **Dieters gulp down:** See Lauren Cooper, "Is a Juice Cleanse Right for You: Cleanse Makers Promise Health and Well-Being in a Bottle. Should You Try One of Them?" *Consumers Report,* March 2016: 19, www.consumerreports.org/diet-nutrition/is-a-juice-cleanse-right-for-you.

Page 16 **Stanley Burroughs was:** See www.wikidoc.org/index.pho/Stanley_Burroughs.

Page 21 **A recent study:** See Mi Joung Kim et al., "Lemon Detox Diet Reduced Body Fat, Insulin Resistance, and Serum hs-CRP Level without Hematological Changes in Overweight Korean Women," *Nutrition Research* 35, no. 5 (May 2015): 409–20, www.ncbi.nlm.nih.gov/pubmed/25912765.

Chapter Three: Diet Nation

Page 25 **In the late 1980s:** See Susan Yager, *The Hundred Year Diet: America's Voracious Appetite for Losing Weight* (New York: Rodale, 2010), 156.

Page 25 **In his slim but prescient volume:** See Carl Malmberg, *Diet and Die* (New York: Hillman-Curl, 1935).

Page 25 **No single subject:** Ibid., 9, 12.

Page 26 **In 1895, Horace Fletcher:** See Horace Fletcher, *Fletcherism What It Is: Or, How I Became Young at Sixty* (New York: Frederick A. Stokes Company, 1913).

Page 27 **Promoted by the slogan:** See Yager, *The Hundred Year Diet*, 12–13. See also Louise Foxcroft, *Calories and Corsets: A History of Dieting over 2000 Years* (London: Profile Books, 2012), 92–95.

Page 28 **A doctor from upstate New York:** See Lisa Breman, "Salisbury Steak: Civil War Health Food," *Smithsonian Magazine*, June 22, 2011, www.smithsonianmag.com/arts-culture/salisbury-steak-civil-war-health-food-18584973.

Page 28 **In his immodestly titled book:** See Malmberg, *Diet and Die*, 92–95.

Page 29 **The notion of separating food groups:** Ibid., 65–77.

Page 29 **the Hollywood diet:** Ibid., 95–101.

Page 31 **George A. Harrop, a respected physician:** Ibid., 101–14.

Page 31 **Even in the late 1800s, John Harvey Kellogg:** See Yager, *The Hundred Year Diet*, 8–10.

Page 32 **the American Tobacco Company:** See Allen M. Brandt, *The Cigarette Century: The Rise, Fall, and Deadly Persistence of the Product that Defined America* (New York: Basic Books, 2007), 71.

Page 32 **My businessman father:** See Gardiner Jameson and Elliott Williams, *The Drinking Man's Diet* (Petaluma, CA: Cameron, 1964).

Page 33 **Did you ever hear of a diet:** Ibid., 5.

Chapter Four: There Are Only Three Diets

Page 36 **during a debate broadcast on CNN:** See "Food Fight: USDA Hosts Heated Forum on Weight Loss Programs," CNN Today, February 24, 2000, transcripts.cnn.com/TRANSCRIPTS/0002/24/tod.08.html.

Page 36 **Carl Malmberg predicted:** See Malmberg, *Diet and Die,* 66.

Page 36 **Jack Sprat first appeared:** See Yager, *The Hundred Year Diet*, 3–6.

Page 39 **But Graham-ism survived:** Ibid., 6–10. See also Harvey Levenstein, *Fear of Food: A History of Why We Worry about What We Eat* (Chicago: The University of Chicago Press, 2012), 36–37.

Page 40 **William Banting, a retired English coffin maker:** See Louise Foxcroft, *Calories and Corsets*, 74–77. See also Gary Taubes, *Good Calories, Bad Calories: Fats, Carbs, and the Controversial Science of Diet and Health* (New York: Alfred A. Knopf, 2007), ix–xii.

Page 43 **To spread the good news:** See William Banting, *Letter on Corpulence Addressed to the Public* (London: Haerison, 1864).

Page 44 **The word *calorie* was nearly unheard of:** See Yager, *The Hundred Year Diet,* 16.

Page 44 **An American chemist named Wilbur Olin Atwater:** See Chin Jou, "Counting Calories," *Distillations,* April 8, 2011, www.sciencehistory.org/distillations/counting-calories.

Page 45 **A California doctor named Lulu Hunt Peters:** See Lulu Hunt Peters, *Diet and Health with Key to the Calories* (Chicago: Reilly and Lee, 1918).

Page 48 **But one long-term study:** See Frank M. Sacks et al., "Comparison of Weight-Loss Diets with Different Compositions of Fat, Protein, and Carbohydrates," *New England Journal of Medicine* 360, no. 9 (February 26, 2009): 859–73, www.nejm.org/doi/full/10.1056/NEJMoa0804748.

Page 50 **"These results show":** See Todd Datz,"Calorie Reduction Key to Weight Loss, Not Food Type," *Harvard Gazette,* February 26, 2009, news.harvard.edu/gazette/story/2009/02/calorie-reduction-key-to-weight-loss-not-food-type/4796.

Chapter Five: Dean Cuisine

Page 51 **a summit in Boston:** See Oldways Common Ground, "Consensus Statement," oldwayspt.org/programs/oldways-common-ground/oldways-common-ground-consensus.

Page 53 **Ornish has positioned himself:** See Dean Ornish, *Stress, Diet, and Your Heart* (New York: Penguin Group, 1982).

Page 54 **As a student at the Baylor College of Medicine:** See Preventive Medicine Research Institute, "Our Team," pmri.org/about/our-team.

Page 64 **A retired San Francisco restaurant owner named Mel Lefer:** See Preventative Medicine Research Institute, "Participant Stories," www.ornish.com/participant-stories/escapefire-testimonial.

Page 64 **Taubes subsequently detailed his message:** See Gary Taubes, *Good Calories, Bad Calories: Fats, Carbs, and the Controversial Science of Diet and Health* (New York: Alfred A. Knopf, 2007), 62.

Page 65 **Taubes went so far as to suggest:** Ibid., 173.

Page 65 **A low point for Ornish:** See Melinda Wenner Moyer and Dean Ornish, "Why Almost Everything Dean Ornish Says about Nutrition is Wrong. Updated with Dean Ornish's Response," *Scientific American*, June 1, 2015, www.scientificamerican.com/article/why-almost-everything-dean-ornish-says-about-nutrition-is-wrong/.

Page 68 **Ornish gained some major allies:** See Caldwell B. Esselstyn, *Prevent and Reverse Heart Disease: The Revolutionary, Scientifically Proven, Nutrition-Based Cure* (New York: Penguin Group, 2007).

Page 72 **China-Oxford-Cornell Study:** See T. Colin Campbell and Thomas M. Campbell, *The China Study: The Most Comprehensive Study of Nutrition Ever Conducted.* (Dallas, TX: BenBella Books, 2005).

Page 73 **In 2005, Ornish partnered with Dr. Peter Carroll:** See Dean Ornish et al., "Intensive Lifestyle Changes May Affect the Progression of Prostate Cancer," *Journal of Urology*, 174, no. 3 (September 2005): 106–70, www.ncbi .nlm.nih.gov/pubmed/16094059.

Page 74 **Ornish and Dr. Elizabeth Blackburn:** See Dean Ornish et al., "Effect of Comprehensive Lifestyle Changes on Telomerase Activity and Telomere Length in Men with Biopsy-Proven Low-Risk Prcstate Cancer: Year Follow-Up of a Descriptive Pilot Study," *Lancet* 14, no.11 (October 1, 2013): 1112–20, www.thelancet.com/journals/lanonc/ articlePIIS1470-(13)70366-8/fulltext.

Page 74 **recipes that Ornish includes in his books:** See Ornish, *Stress, Diet, and Your Heart*, 343–42. See also Dean Ornish, *The Spectrum: A Scientifically Proven Program to Feel Better, Live Longer, Lose Weight, Gain Health* (New York: Ballantine Books, 2007), 239–340.

Chapter Six: Low-Carb Country

Page 79 **Agatston's work resulted in numerous scientific papers:** See Axel Schmermund, "The Agatston Calcium Score: A Milestone in the History of Cardiac CT," *Journal* *of Cardiovascular Tomography* 8 (2014): 414–17, www.journalofcardiovascularct.com/article/S1934-5925(14)00248-2/abstract.

Page 81 **insisted the program needed a catchier name:** See Arthur Agatston, *The South Beach Diet: The Delicious, Doctor-Designed, Foolproof Plan for Fast and Healthy Weight Loss* (New York: Rodale, 2003).

Page 81 **In 2015, Nutrisystem, Inc.:** See Nutrisystem News Room, "Nutrisystem, Inc. Acquired South Beach Diet Brand from SBD Holdings Group" (press release), newsroom.nutrisystem.com/nutrisystem-inc-acquires-south-beach-diet-brand-from-sbd-holdings-group-corp/.

Page 83 **nearly half of the recommended daily requirement:** See American Heart Association, "Whole Grains, Refined Grains, and Dietary Fiber," www.heart.org/en/healthy-living/healthy-eating/eat-smart/nutrition-basics/whole-grains-refined-grains-and-dietary-fiber.

Page 85 **It's easy to understand:** See Robert C. Atkins, *Dr. Atkins' Diet Revolution: The High-Calorie Way to Stay Thin Forever* (New York: Bantam, 1972), 7.

Page 85 **"carbohydrate poisoning":** Ibid., 3.

Page 86 **The U.S. Dietary Guidelines:** See U.S. Department of Health and Human Services and U.S. Department of Agriculture, *2015–2020 Dietary Guidelines for Americans*, 8th edition, 2015, 97, https://www.dietaryguidelines.gov/current-dietary-guidelines/2015-2020-dietary-guidelines.

Page 86 **claiming that followers:** See Atkins, *Dr. Atkins' Diet Revolution: The High-Calorie Way to Stay Thin Forever*, 3.

Page 86 **you can replace the steak:** Ibid., 132.

Page 86–88 **One participant routinely had:** Ibid., 39.

Page 88 **In a 2003 study of fifty-three obese women:** See Bonnie Brehm et al., "A Randomized Trial Comparing a Very Low Carbohydrate Diet and a Calorie-Restricted Low Fat Diet on Body Weight and Cardiovascular Risk Factors in Healthy Women," *Journal of Endocrinol Metabolism* 88, no.4 (April 2003): 1617–23, www.ncbi.nlm.nih.gov/pubmed/12679447.

Page 88 **A subsequent study:** See Alain Nordmann et al., "Effects of Low-Carbohydrate vs Low-Fat Diets on Weight Loss and Cardiovascular Risk Factors: A Meta-Analysis of Randomized Controlled Trials," *Archives of Internal Medicine* 166, no. 3 (February 13, 2006): 285–93, www.ncbi.nlm.nih.gov/pubmed/16476868.

Page 89 **Polish nutritionist Maciej Banach:** Maciej Banach presented his findings in a talk titled "Low Carbohydrate Diets Are Unsafe and Should Be Avoided" at a meeting of the European Society of Cardiology on August 18, 2018, www.escardio.org/The-ESC/Press-Office/Press-releases/Low-carbohydrate-diets-are-unsafe-and-should-be-avoided.

Page 89 **Alas, Atkins' final years:** See N. R. Kleinfield, "Just What Killed the Diet Doctor, and What Keeps the Issue Alive?" The *New York Times*, February 11, 2004, www.nytimes.com/2004/02/11/nyregion/just-what-killed-the-diet-doctor-and-what-keeps-the-issue-alive.html. See also Douglas Martin, "Dr. Robert C. Atkins, Author of Controversial Best-Selling Diet Books, Is Dead at 72," *New York Times*, April 18, 2003, www.nytimes.com/2003/04/18/nyregion/dr-robert-c-atkins-author-controversial-but-bestselling-diet-books-dead-72.html. See also Melanie Warner, Atkins, the Diet Company, Seeks Protection from Its Creditors," *New York Times*, August, 1, 2005, www.nytimes.com/2005/08/01/business/atkins-the-diet-company-seeks-protection-from-its-creditors.html.

Page 89 **Atkins' legacy remains alive and well:** See S. Boyd Eaton, Melvin Konner.

Page 91 **he told a conference of prominent nutritionists:** The conference, organized by Oldways in Boston, took place between November 16 and 18, 2015.

Page 91 **"We traditionally divide our foods into four basic groups":** See S. Boyd Eaton, Marjorie Shostak, Melvin Konner, *The Paleolithic Prescription: A Program of Diet and Exercise and a Design for Living* (New York: Harper and Row, 1988), 83.

Page 92 **"Paleolithic prescription":** Ibid., 275–76.

Page 92 **six simple rules:** See Loren Cordain, *The Paleo Diet: Lose Weight and Get Healthy by Eating the Foods You Were Designed to Eat* (Boston: Houghton Mifflin Harcourt, 2002), 23.

Page 93 **a blink of the evolutionary eye:** See Eaton, *The Paleolithic Prescription: A Program of Diet and Exercise and a Design for Living*, 26.

Page 93 **"Has no basis in archaeological reality":** Warriner said this during a TEDx talk in January 2013, "Debunking the Paleo Diet," www.youtube.com/watch?v=BMOjVYgYaG8.

Page 94 **the genes that served ancient humans:** See Marlene Zuk, *Paleofantasy: What Evolution Really Tells Us About Sex, Diet, and How We Live* (New York: W.W. Norton, 2013), 6.

Page 95 **In his seminal book, Atkins described:** See Atkins, *Dr. Atkins' Diet Revolution: The High-Calorie Way to Stay Thin Forever*, 12.

Page 96 **keto diets call for between:** See U. S. Department of Health and Human Services and U.S. Department of Agriculture, *2015–2020 Dietary Guidelines for Americans*, 8th edition, 2015, 97, www.dietaryguidelines.gov/current-dietary-guidelines/2015-2020-dietary-guidelines.

Page 96 **we're talking about eating fat:** See Leanne Vogel, *The Keto Diet: The Complete Guide to a High-Fat Diet* (Las Vegas: Victory Bell Publishing, 2017), 50–51.

Page 96 **examined the results of numerous studies:** See Christophe Kosinski and François R. Jornayvaz, "Effects of Ketogenic Diets on Cardiovascular Risk Factors: Evidence from Animal and Human Studies," *Nutrients* 9, no. 5 (May 19, 2017): 517, www.mdpi.com/2072-6643/9/5/517.

Page 99 **he is also an accidental, accidental gluten-free diet doctor:** See Arthur Agatston, *The South Beach Diet Gluten Solution: The Delicious, Doctor-Designed, Gluten-Aware Plan for Losing Weight and Feeling Great—Fast!* (New York: Rodale, 2013).

Chapter Seven: Losers Pay

Page 102 **Oprah Winfrey, perhaps the world's most famous:** See Leslie Picker, "Shares of Weight Watchers Jump as Oprah Winfrey Takes a Stake," *New York Times*, October 19, 2015, www.nytimes.com/2015/10/20/business/dealbook/shares-of-weight-watchers-jump-as-oprah-winfrey-takes-a-stake.html.

Page 105 **By attending those WW meetings:** See Jean Nidetch, *The Story of Weight Watchers* (New York: W/W Twentyfirst, 1970).

Page 106 **I dieted in preparation for birthday parties:** Ibid., 14.

Page 112 **In the late 1970s, the firm, having been sold:** See Robert J. Cole, "H.J. Heintz to Buy Weight Watchers for $71 Million," *New York Times*, May 5, 1978, www.nytimes.com/1978/05/05/archives/hj-heinz-to-buy-weight-watchers-for-71-million-hj-heinz-agrees-to.html.

Page 112 **Weight Watchers changed its name:** See Micah Maidenberg, "Weight Watchers Changes Name As It Shifts Mission," *Wall Street Journal*, September 24, 2018, www.wsj.com/articles/weight-watchers-changes-name-as-it-shifts-mission-1537807754.

Page 113 **WW has been a repeat winner:** See U. S. News Staff, "U. S. News Best 35 Diets Overall," U. S. News & World Report, January 2, 2020, health.usnews.com/wellness/food/slideshows/best-diets-overall.

Page 119 **WW members dropped more weight:** See Craig A. Johnson et al., "A Randomized Controlled Trial of a Community-Based Behavioral Counseling Program," *American Journal of Medicine* 126, no. 12 (December 2013): 19–24, www.ncbi.nlm.nih.gov/pubmed/24135513.

Page 119 **the company commissioned a six-month clinical trial:** See Deborah Tate, "Evaluation of a Commercial Program on Weight Loss and Health Outcomes," U. S. National Library of Medicine, clinicaltrials.gov/ct2/show/NCT03037567.

Chapter Eight: Hill Tribe

Page 124 ***Newsweek* published an infographic:** See *Newsweek*, April 15, 2011, www.asabbathblog.com/2011/04/newsweek-magazine-says-be-adventist-if.html.

Page 124 **That is an understatement:** See Dan Buettner, *The Blue Zones: 9 Lessons for Living Longer from the People Who've Lived the Longest* (Washington, DC: The National Geographic Society, 2008): 123–64.

Page 125 **When Professor Rhonda Spencer-Hwang:** See Rhonda Spencer-Hwang et al. "Adverse Childhood Experiences among a Community of Resilient Centenarians and Seniors: Implications for a Chronic

Disease Prevention Framework," *Permanente Journal* 22, (March 2018): 17–146, www.ncbi.nlm.nih.gov/pubmed/29702049.

Page 126 **With origins that date back seven decades:** See Adventist Health Study website: adventisthealthstudy.org/?rsource=publichealth.llu.edu/adventist-health-studies.

Page 126 **The origins of the Adventist study:** See Ansel Oliver, "Loma Linda's Longevity Legacy," *Scope*, Spring 2018, issuu.com/lluh/docs/2018-spring-scope.

Page 128 **one that would have strained:** See Emilo Ros, "Health Benefits of Nut Consumption", *Nutrients* 2, no. 7 (July 2010): 652–82.

Page 132 **In an independent examination:** See Walter Willett, "Lessons from Dietary Studies in Adventists and Questions for the Future," *American Journal of Clinical Nutrition* 78 no. 3 (September 2003): 539S—43S, academic.oup.com/ajcn/article/78/3/539S/4689994.

Chapter Nine: Club Med

Page 138 **One massive study:** See Antonia Trichopoulou et al., "Modified Mediterranean Diet and Survival: EPIC Elderly Prospective Cohort Study," *BMJ* 330 (April 28, 2005): 991–98, www.ncbi.nlm.nih.gov/pmc/articles/PMC557144.

Page 138 **adopting a Mediterranean diet:** See Ramón Estruch et al., "Primary Prevention of Cardiovascular Disease with a Mediterranean Diet," *New England Journal of Medicine* 368 (April 4, 2013): 1279–90, www.nejm.org/doi/full/10.1056/NEJMoa1200303?query=featured_home#t=article.

Page 139 **at times, controversial:** See Jane E. Brody, "Dr. Ancel Keys, 100, Promoter of Mediterranean Diet, Dies," *The New York Times*, November 23, 2004, www.nytimes.com/2004/11/23/obituaries/dr-ancel-keys-100-promoter-of-mediterranean-diet-dies.html.

Page 140 **Seven Countries Study:** See Katherine Pett et al., "Ancel Keys and the Seven Countries Study: An Evidence-Based Response to Revisionist Histories," The True Health Initiative, August 1, 2017, www.truehealthinitiative.org/wp-content/uploads/2017/07/SCS-White-Paper.THI_.8-1-17.pdf.

Page 142 **Oldways Preservation Trust:** See Nina Teicholz, *The Big Fat Surprise: Why Butter, Meat, and Cheese Belong in a Healthy Diet* (New York: Simon and Schuster, 2014): 183–97.

Page 143 **more than seven thousand university students:** See Maria Bes-Rastrollo et al., "Olive Oil Consumption and Weight Change: The SUN Prospective Cohort Study," *Lipids* 41, no. 3 (March 2006), www.ncbi.nlm.nih.gov/pubmed/16711599.

Page 144 **vegetables, seeds, and legumes are good sources of flavonoids:** See Effie Vasilopoulou et al., "The Antioxidant Properties of Greek Foods and the Flavonoid Content of the Mediterranean Menu," *Current Medicinal Chemistry* 5, no. 1 (February 2005): 33–45.

Page 146 **they no longer ate a Mediterranean diet:** See Caitlin Dewey, "Mediterranean Children Stopped Eating the Mediterranean Diet, and They Now Have the Highest Obesity Rates in Europe," The *Washington Post*, May 30, 2018, https://www.washingtonpost.com/news/wonk/wp/2018/05/30/mediterranean-children-stopped-eating-the-mediterranean-diet-and-they-now-have-the-highest-obesity-rates-in-europe.

Chapter Ten: A French Connection

Page 148 **the French consume some of the tastiest food:** See Jean Ferrières, "The French Paradox: Lessons for Other Countries," *Heart* 90, (January 2004): 107–11, www.ncbi.nlm.nih.gov/pmc/articles/PMC1768013.

Page 148 **Still, the French maintain low rates of obesity:** See Bradley Sawyer and Daniel McDermott, "How Do Mortality Rates in the U.S. Compare to Other Countries?" Health System Tracker, February 14, 2019, www.healthsystemtracker.org/chart-collection/mortality-rates-u-s-compare-countries/#item-start.

Page 148 **While four in ten Americans:** See Organization for Economic Cooperation and Development, "Obesity Update" 2017, www.oecd.org/health/obesity-update.htm.

Page 154 **Paul Rozin, a psychologist at the University of Pennsylvania:** See Paul Rozin, Abigail K. Remick, Claude Fischler, "Broad Themes of Difference between French and Americans in Attitudes to Food and Other Life Domains: Personal Versus Communal Values, Quality Versus Quantity, and Comforts Versus Joys," *Frontiers in Psychology* 177 no. 2 (July 2011): 177, www.ncbi.nlm.nih .gov/pmc/articles/PMC3145256.

Page 157 **some straightforward rules that Guiliano sets out:** See Mirielle Guiliano, *French Women Don't Get Fat: The Secret of Eating for Pleasure* (New York: Alfred A. Knopf, 2005), 254–55.

Chapter Eleven: The Reckoning

Page 163 **Demonstrating that all calories aren't created equal:** See Cara Ebbeling et al., "Effects of Dietary Composition on Energy Expenditure during Weight-loss Maintenance," *Journal of the American Medical Association* 307, no. 24 (June 27, 2012), www.ncbi.nlm.nih.gov/ pubmed/22735432.

Page 164 **A group of adolescent boys:** See David Ludwig et al., "High Glycemic Index Foods, Overeating, and Obesity," *Pediatrics* 103, no. 3 (March 1999): E26, www.ncbi.nlm.nih .gov/pubmed/10049982.

Pages 164–165 **activate the same brain pathways as addictive drugs:** See Joan Ifland et al., "Refined Food Addiction: A Classic Substance Abuse Disorder," *Medical Hypotheses* 72, no. 5 (May 2009): 518–26, www.ncbi.nlm.nih.gov/ pubmed/19223127.

Page 165 **Harvard anthropologist Vilhjalmur Stefansson:** See Gary Taubes, *Good Calories, Bad Calories: Fats, Carbs, and the Controversial Science of Diet and Health* (New York: Alfred A. Knopf, 2007), 320–24.

Page 166 **Yudkin pulled no punches:** See John Yudkin, *Pure, White, and Deadly: How Sugar Is Killing Us and What We Can Do to Stop It* (London: Viking, 1986), 167.

Page 166 **he could make two statements:** Ibid, 2–3.

Page 168 **cane in its just-harvested state:** See Food and Agriculture Organization of the United Nations, Definition and Classification of Commodities (Draft) Sugar Crops and Sweeteners, www.fao.org/es/faodef/fdef03e.HTM.

Page 169 **that Americans satisfied their appetite:** See Sidney A. Mintz, *Sweetness and Power: The Place of Sugar in Modern History* (New York: Viking Penguin, 1985), 198–99.

Page 169 **Things got a lot worse:** See Stephan Guyenet, "By 2026, the US Diet Will Be 100 Percent Sugar" *Whole Health Source,* February 18, 2012, wholehealthsource.blogspot .com/2012/02/by-2606-us-diet-will-be-100-percent.html.

Page 172 **a conflicting body of research:** See Susan E. Swithers, "Artificial Sweeteners Produce the Counterintuitive Effect of Inducing Metabolic Derangements," *Trends in Endocrinology & Metabolism* 24, no. 9 (September 2013): 431–41, www.ncbi.nlm.nih.gov/pubmed/23850261.

Page 172 **M. Yanina Pepino, of the University of Illinois:** See M. Yanina Pepino et al., "Sucralose Affects Glycemic and Hormonal Responses to an Oral Glucose Load," *Diabetes Care* 36, no. 9 (September 2013): 2530–35, care.diabetesjournals.org/content/early/2013/04/30/dc12-2221.

Page 172 **a group of Australian researchers:** See Qiao-Ping Wang et al. "Sucralose Promotes Food Intake Through NPY and a Neuronal Fasting Response," *Cell Metabolism* 24, no. 1 (July 12, 2016): 75–90, www.cell.com/cell-metabolism/fulltext/S1550-4131(16)30296-0?_returnURL=https%3A%2F%2Flinkinghub.elsevier.com%2Fretrieve%2Fpii%2FS1550413116302960%3Fshowall%3Dtrue.

Page 173 **the average American gulps:** See Grace Youn, "Daily Sugar Intake," *The Nightingale*, February 20, 2019, www.angelesinstitute.edu/thenightingale/daily-sugar-intake.

Page 173 **Lustig told me to beware of the following:** See Robert H. Lustig, *Fat Chance: Beating the Odds Against Sugar, Processed Food, Obesity and Disease* (New York: Hudson Street Press, 2013), 196.

Page 175 **As Yudkin asserted:** See John Yudkin, *Pure, White, and Deadly: How Sugar is Killing Us and What We Can Do to Stop It*, 70.

Page 177 **consumed at least 400 calories more:** See Rosalind A. Breslow, "Diets of Drinkers on Drinking and Nondrinking Days: NHANES 2003–2008," *American Journal of Clinical Nutrition* 97, no. 5 (May 1, 2013): 1068–75, academic.oup.com/ajcn/article/97/5/1068/4577068.

Page 178 **alcohol stimulated the same brain cells:** See Sarah Cains et al., "Agrp Neuron Activity Is Required for Alcohol-Induced Overeating," *Nature Communications* 8, no. 14014 (January 10, 2017), www.nature.com/articles/ncomms14014.

Page 178 **metabolisms plummet by as much as 73 percent:** See Scott Q. Siler, Richard N., Neese and Marc K. Hellerstein, "De Novo Lipogenesis, Lipid Kinetics, and Whole-Body Lipid Balances in Humans after Acute Alcohol Consumption," *American Journal of Clinical Nutrition* 70, no. 5 (November 1999): 928–36, academic.oup.com/ajcn/article/70/5/928/4729236.

Page 179 **a group of young men:** See Arlet V. Nedeltcheva et al., "Insufficient Sleep Undermines Dietary Efforts to Reduce Adiposity," *Annals of Internal Medicine* 153, no. 7 (October 5, 2010): 435–41, www.annals.org/aim/fullarticle/doi/10.7326/0003-4819-153-7-201010050-00006.

Page 179 **men ate between 385 and 560 calories:** See H. K. Al Khatib, S. V. Harding, and J. Darzi and G. K. Pot, "The Effects of Partial Sleep Deprivation on Energy Balance: A Systematic Review and Meta-Analysis," *European Journal of Clinical Nutrition* 71 (November 2, 2016): 614–24, www.nature.com/articles/ejcn2016201.

Page 180 **the operative word here is *moderate*:** See "Alcohol Use: Weighing Risks and Benefits," *Mayo Clinic Healthy Lifestyle: Nutrition and Healthy Eating*, www.mayoclinic.org/healthy-lifestyle/nutrition-and-healthy-eating/in-depth/alcohol/art-20044551.

Page 180 **"several kilograms":** See Tavia Gordon and William B. Kannel, "Drinking and Its Relation to Smoking, BP, Blood Lipids, and Uric Acid," *Archives of Internal Medicine* 143, no. 7 (July 1983): 1366–74, jamanetwork.com/journals/jamainternalmedicine/article-abstract/603361.

Chapter Twelve: Big Winners

Page 182 **National Weight Control Registry:** See the National Weight Control Registry website, www.nwcr.ws.

Page 184 **"Who better to tell you how to lose weight":** See Anne M. Fletcher, *Thin for Life: Ten Keys to Success from People Who Have Lost Weight and Kept It Off* (Shelburne, VT: Chapters Publishing, 1994), 13.

Page 184 **the secret to weight loss is there is no single secret:** See Ibid., 61.

BIBLIOGRAPHY

Aamodt, Sandra. *Why Diets Make Us Fat: The Unintended Consequences of Our Obsession with Weight Loss.* New York: Current, 2016.

Ades, Phillip A., and the editors of *Eating Well. Eating Well for a Healthy Heart Cookbook: A Cardiologist's Guide to Adding Years to Your Life.* Woodstock, VT: Countryman Press, 2008.

Agatston, Arthur. *The South Beach Diet: The Delicious, Doctor-Designed, Fool-Proof Plan for Fast and Healthy Weight Loss.* New York: Rodale, 2003.

———. *The South Beach Diet Gluten Solution: The Delicious, Doctor-Designed, Gluten-Aware Plan for Losing Weight and Feeling Great—Fast!* New York: Rodale, 2013.

———. *The South Beach Wake-Up Call: Why America is Getting Still Fatter and Sicker.* New York: Rodale, 2011.

Atkins, Robert C. *Dr. Atkins' Diet Revolution: The High-Calorie Way to Stay Thin Forever.* New York: Bantam, 1972.

Babor, Thomas, et al. *Alcohol: No Ordinary Commodity.* Oxford: Oxford University Press, 2003.

Banting, William. *Letter on Corpulence Addressed to the Public.* London: Haerison, 1864.

Berland, Mike. *Become a Fat-Burning Machine: The 12-Week Diet.* New York: Regan Arts, 2015.

Blaser, Martin J. *Missing Microbes: How the Overuse of Antibiotics Is Fueling Our Modern Plagues.* New York: Henry Holt, 2014.

Bobrow-Strain, Aaron. *White Bread: A Social History of the Store-Bought Loaf.* Boston: Beacon Press, 2012.

Brandt, Allen M. *The Cigarette Century: The Rise, Fall, and Deadly Persistence of the Product that Defined America.* New York: Basic Books, 2007.

Buettner, Dan. *The Blue Zones: 9 Lessons for Living Longer from the People Who've Lived the Longest.* Washington, DC: National Geographic Society, 2008.

Burroughs, Stanley A. *The Master Cleanser.* Riverside, CA: Burroughs Books, 1976.

Campbell, T. Colin and Thomas M. Campbell. *The China Study: The Most Comprehensive Study of Nutrition Ever Conducted.* Dallas, TX: BenBella Books, 2005.

Campbell, T. Colin and Howard Jacobson. *The Low-Carb Fraud.* Dallas, TX: BenBella Books, 2014.

Cordain, Loren. *The Paleo Diet: Lose Weight and Get Healthy by Eating the Foods You Were Designed to Eat.* Boston: Houghton Mifflin Harcourt, 2002.

Cornaro, Luigi. *The Art of Living Long.* Milwaukee, WI: William F. Butler, 1917.

Davis, William. *Wheat Belly: Lose the Wheat, Lose the Weight, and Find Your Path Back to Health.* New York: Rodale, 2011.

Duncan, T. C. *How to Become Plump.* Chicago: Duncan Brothers, 1878.

Eaton, S. Boyd, Marjorie Shostak, and Melvin Konner. *The Paleolithic Prescription: A Program of Diet and Exercise and a Design for Living.* New York; Harper and Row, 1988.

Egan, Sophie. *Devoured: How What We Eat Defines Who We Are.* New York: Harper Collins, 2016.

Esselstyn, Caldwell B. *Prevent and Reverse Heart Disease: The Revolutionary, Scientifically Proven, Nutrition-Based Cure.* New York: Avery, 2007.

Feinman, Richard David. *Nutrition in Crisis: Flawed Studies, Misleading Advice, and the Real Science of Human Metabolism.* White River Junction, VT: Chelsea Green, 2019.

Fischler, Claude and Estelle Masson. *Manger: Français, Européans et Américains Face à L'Alimentation.* Paris: Odile Jacob, 2008.

Fletcher, Anne M. *Thin for Life: Ten Keys to Success from People Who Have Lost Weight and Kept It Off.* Shelburne, VT: Chapters, 1994.

Fletcher, Horace A. M. *Fletcherism, What It Is: Or, How I Became Young at Sixty.* New York: Frederick A. Stokes, 1913.

Foxcroft, Louise. *Calories and Corsets: A History of Dieting over 2,000 Years.* London: Profile Books, 2012.

Freedhoff, Yoni. *The Diet Fix: Why Diets Fail and How to Make Yours Work.* New York: Harmony Books, 2014.

Greenberg, Paul *The Omega Principle: Seafood and the Quest for a Long Life and a Healthier Planet.* New York: Penguin Press, 2018.

Guiliano, Mireille. *French Women Don't Get Fat: The Secret of Eating for Pleasure.* New York: Alfred A. Knopf, 2005.

Harrington, Rebecca. *I'll Have What She's Having: My Adventures in Celebrity Dining.* New York: Vintage Books, 2015.

Harrison, Christy. *Anti-Diet: Reclaim Your Time, Money, Well-Being, and Happiness Through Intuitive Eating.* New York: Little, Brown Spark, 2019.

Hartwig, Dallas and Melissa. *It Starts with Food: Discover the Whole30 and Change Your Life in Unexpected Ways.* Las Vegas: Victory Belt, 2012.

Heller, Marla. *The Dash Diet Weight Loss Solution: Two Weeks to Drop Pounds, Boost Metabolism, and Get Healthy.* New York: Grand Central, 2012.

Hyman, Mark. *The Blood Sugar Solution: The Ultrahealthy Program for Losing Weight, Preventing Disease, and Feeling Great Now!* New York: Little Brown, 2012.

Jameson, Gardiner and Elliott Williams. *The Drinking Man's Diet.* Petaluma, CA: Cameron, 1964.

Kaminsky, Peter. *Culinary Intelligence: The Art of Eating Healthy (and Really Well).* New York: Alfred A. Knopf, 2012.

Kamp, David. *The United States of Arugula: How We Became a Gourmet Nation.* New York: Broadway Books, 2006.

Kessler, David A. *The End of Overeating: Taking Control of the Insatiable American Appetite.* New York: Rodale, 2009.

Keys, Ancel and Margaret Keys. *Eat Well and Stay Well.* Garden City, NY: Doubleday, 1959.

Kremezi, Aglaia. *Foods of the Greek Islands: Cooking and Culture at the Crossroads of the Mediterranean.* Boston: Houghton Mifflin, 2000.

Leighton, H. Stewart, Morrison C. Bethea, Sam S. Andrews, and Luis A. Balart. *The New Sugar Busters: Cut Sugar to Trim Fat.* New York: Ballantine Books, 2003.

Levenstein, Harvey. *Fear of Food: A History of Why We Worry about What We Eat.* Chicago: The University of Chicago Press, 2012.

———. *Paradox of Plenty: A Social History of Eating In Modern America.* Berkeley, CA: University of California Press, 2003.

———. *Revolution at the Table: The Transformation of the American Diet.* Berkeley, CA: The University of California Press, 2003.

Ludwig. David. *Always Hungry? Conquer Cravings, Retrain Your Fat Cells, and Lose Weight Permanently.* New York: Grand Central, 2016.

Lustig, Robert H. *Fat Chance: Beating the Odds Against Sugar, Processed Food, Obesity and Disease.* New York: Hudson Street Press, 2013,

Malmberg, Carl. *Diet and Die.* New York: Hillman-Curl, 1935.

Mann, Traci. *Secrets from the Eating Lab: The Science of Weight Loss, the Myth of Willpower, and Why You Should Never Diet Again.* New York: HarperCollins, 2015.

Mayer, Jean. *Overweight: Causes, Costs, and Control.* Englewood Cliffs, NJ: Prentice Hall, 1968.

McQuaid, John. *Tasty: The Art and Science of What We Eat.* New York: Scribner, 2015.

Mintz, Sidney W. *Sweetness and Power: The Place of Sugar in Modern History.* New York: Viking Penguin, 1985.

———. *Tasting Food, Tasting Freedom: Excursions into Eating, Culture, and the Past.* Boston: Beacon Press, 1996.

Moss, Michael, *Salt Sugar Fat: How the Food Giants Hooked Us.* New York: Random House, 2013

Nestle, Marion. *Food Politics: How the Food Industry Influences Nutrition and Health.* Berkeley, CA: University of California Press, 2007.

Nidetch, Jean. *The Story of Weight Watchers.* New York: W/W Twentyfirst, 1970.

Olmstead, Larry. *Real Food Fake Food: Why You Don't Know What You're Eating and What You Can Do About It.* Chapel Hill, NC: Algonquin Books of Chapel Hill, 2016.

Ornish, Dean. *Dr. Dean Ornish's Program for Reversing Heart Disease: The Only System Scientifically Proven to Reverse Heart Disease Without Drugs or Surgery.* New York: Random House, 1990.

———. *The Spectrum: A Scientifically Proven Program to Feel Better, Live Longer, Lose Weight, Gain Health.* New York: Ballantine Books, 2007.

———. *Stress, Diet, and Your Heart.* New York: Penguin Group, 1982.

Ozner, Michael. *The Complete Mediterranean Diet: Everything You Need to Know to Lose Weight and Lower Your Risk of Heart Disease.* Dallas, TX: BenBella Books, 2014.

Pépin, Jacques. *The Apprentice: My Life in the Kitchen.* Boston: Houghton Mifflin Harcourt, 2003.

Perlmutter, David with Kristin Loberg. *Grain Brain: The Surprising Truth about Wheat, Carbs, and Sugar—Your Brain's Silent Killers.* New York: Little Brown, 2013.

Peters, Lulu Hunt. *Diet and Health with Key to the Calories.* Chicago: Reilly and Lee, 1918.

Polivy, Janet and C. Peter Herman. *Breaking the Diet Habit: The Natural Weight Alternative.* New York: Basic Books, 1983.

Pollan, Michael. *In Defense of Food: An Eater's Manifesto.* New York: Penguin Press, 2008.

Pulde, Alona and Mathew Lederman. *The Forks Over Knives Plan: A 4-Week Meal by-Meal Makeover.* New York: Touchstone, 2014.

Ramos, Amy. *The Complete Ketogenic Diet for Beginners: Your Essential Guide to Living the Keto Lifestyle.* Berkeley, CA: Rockridge Press, 2016.

Roach, Mary. *Gulp: Adventures on the Alimentary Canal.* New York: W.W. Norton, 2013

Roizen, Michael F. and Mehmet C. Oz. *You on a Diet: The Owner's Manual for Waist Management.* New York: Free Press, 2006.

Roth, J. D. *The Big Fat Truth: Behind the Scenes Secrets to Losing Weight and Gaining the Inner Strength to Transform Your Life.* New York: Reader's Digest, 2016.

Sax, David. *The Tastemakers: A Celebrity Rice Farmer, a Food Truck Lobbyist, and Other Trends on Your Plate.* New York: PublicAffairs, 2014.

Schatzker, Mark. *The Dorito Effect: The Surprising Truth About Food and Flavor. New York:* Simon and Schuster, 2015.

Shanahan, Catherine with Luke Shanahan. *Deep Nutrition: Why Your Genes Need Traditional Food.* New York: Flatiron Books, 2016.

Smil, Vaclav. *Should We Eat Meat? Evolution and Consequences of Modern Carnivory.* Oxford, UK: John Wiley and Sons, 2013.

Tara, Sylvia. *The Secret Life of Fat: The Science Behind the Body's Least Understood Organ and What It Means for You.* New York: W.W. Norton, 2017.

Taubes, Gary. *The Case Against Sugar.* New York: Knopf, 2016.

———. *Good Calories, Bad Calories: Fats, Carbs, and the Controversial Science of Diet and Health.* New York: Alfred A. Knopf, 2007.

———. *Why We Get Fat and What to Do About It.* New York: Alfred A. Knopf, 2011.

Teicholz, Nina. *The Big Fat Surprise: Why Butter, Meat, and Cheese Belong in a Healthy Diet.* New York: Simon and Schuster, 2014.

Thomas, Laura. *Just Eat: How Intuitive Eating Can Help You Get Your Shit Together Around Food.* London: Bluebird, 2019.

United States Department of Agriculture, *Dietary Guidelines for Americans 2015–2020.* New York: Skyhorse Publishing, 2017.

Urban, Melissa Hartwig and Dallas Hartwig. *The Whole30: The 30-Day Guide to Total Health and Food Freedom.* Boston: Houghton Mifflin Harcourt, 2015.

Vogel, Leanne. *The Keto Diet: The Complete Guide to a High-Fat Diet.* Las Vegas: Victory Bell Publishing, 2017.

Wansink, Brian. *Mindless Eating: Why We Eat More Than We Think.* New York: Bantam Books, 2006.

Warner, Melanie. *Pandora's Lunchbox: How Processed Food Took Over the American Meal.* New York: Scribner, 2013.

Weeks, John Howard. *The Healthiest People on Earth: Your Guide to Living 10 Years Longer with Adventist Family Secrets and Plant-Based Recipes.* Dallas, TX: BenBella Books, 2018.

Willett, Walter and Patrick J. Skerrett. *Eat, Drink, and Be Healthy: The Harvard Medical School Guide to Healthy Eating.* New York: Free Press, 2017.

Willett, Walter, Malisssa Wood, and Dan Childs. *Thinfluence: Thin-flu-ence (noun) the Powerful and Surprising Effect Friends, Family, Work, and Environment Have on Weight.* New York: Rodale, 2014.

Wrangham, Richard. *Catching Fire: How Cooking Made Us Human.* New York: Basic Books, 2009.

Yager, Susan. *The Hundred Year Diet: America's Voracious Appetite for Losing Weight.* New York: Rodale, 2010.

Yudkin, John. *Pure, White, and Deadly: How Sugar Is Killing Us and What We Can Do to Stop It.* London: Viking, 1986.

Zuk, Marlene. *Paleofantasy: What Evolution Really Tells Us About Sex, Diet, and How We Live.* New York: W.W. Norton, 2013.

ACKNOWLEDGMENTS

A special thanks to Dr. Dennis Beatty whose thoughtful insistence that losing weight might dramatically improve my well-being set me on the journey that led to this book and a slimmer me. Dr. Dennis, you were right. I doubt I would have summoned the willpower to follow the doctor's orders were it not for the inspiration and support (and occasional not-so-subtle reminder) of my three daughters, Robyn, Jillian, and Molly. You have made my life better and, I hope, longer.

I have tremendous respect for the physicians, nutritionists, and scientists who dedicate their careers toward building a greater understanding of the causes and "cures" for obesity, one of our society's most confounding and pervasive medical problems. Thanks to all of you. It is an honor that so many experts, some mentioned by name in this book, others not, took the time to talk with me, a rank amateur, about their life's work. It's a cliché to say that any errors and misinterpretations are completely my own, but I think it bears repeating.

Aglaia Kremezi and Costas Moraitis welcomed me to Kea, the beautiful island they call home, and allowed me to look over their shoulders as they proved that Greek vegetable-based dishes could be tastier and more satisfying than recipes that rely on meat. My only complaint is that now I want to live on Kea forever—and enjoy many more wonderful meals in Aglaia and Costas' shady outdoor kitchen.

No writer could ask for a more stalwart comrade than David Black. I suspect the earnings from my work barely keep his agency in paper clips, but he manages to give the impression that I am his only client. He replies to emails and phone calls at warp speed. He took way more time and was way more diligent shaping the proposal for this book than duty required. Thanks also to Ayla Zuraw-Friedland, Gary Morris, and Sarah Smith at the David Black Agency.

David once again placed a book of mine with the ideal editor. A very special thanks to the terrific Lorena Jones and the crew at Ten Speed Press: designer Isabelle Gioffredi, production designer Mari Gill, production manager Dan Myers, publicist Lauren Kretzchmar, and marketer Brianne Sperber. It's difficult to describe the great respect I have for copy editors. Deborah Kops' eagle eye saved me from embarrassment more times than I want to admit, as did proofreader Andrea Chesman.

As always, I have the advantage on having the world's most wonderful editor, my wife, Rux Martin, on call 24-7. She did yeoman's work on this stubborn manuscript. And, Rux, I'm really sorry I made you taste my buckwheat-noodle dish. They weren't earthworms. Honest.

INDEX

A

Abrams, Steven, 52
Adventist Health Study, 126–28, 132
Agatston, Arthur, 79–85, 87, 97–100, 160, 161, 192
alcohol, 163, 176–80, 195
American approach to eating, 151–54, 156
American Heart Association, 70, 80, 81, 83, 173
American Medical Association, 31
American Tobacco Company, 32
antioxidants, 144
Applegate, Liz, 20–21
Atkins, Robert, 36, 84, 85–86, 88, 89, 95
Atkins' Diet, 12, 42, 43, 46, 85–86, 87, 88, 114
Atwater, Wilbur Olin, 44–45, 198

B

Banach, Maciej, 89
banana and skim milk diet, 31
Banting, William, 40–43, 50, 84, 192, 198
Baylor College of Medicine, 54, 56
beans, 6, 193, 197
Beatty, Dennis, 1–2, 12, 14–15, 80, 159–60, 177, 189–90, 197
Beyoncé, 16
Blackburn, Elizabeth, 74
Blue Apron, 3
Blue Zones, 124, 132
Brehm, Bonnie, 88
Breslow, Rosalind, 177
Brillat-Savarin, Jean Anthelme, 41
Buettner, Dan, 124, 132
Burroughs, Stanley, 16, 18–19

C

cabbage soup diet, 32, 199
calcium, 80, 160
California Pacific Medical Center, 63
calories
  counting, 44–48, 50
  misconception about, 162–63
Cameron, Robert, 32–33, 199
Campbell, T. Colin, 40, 71–72, 78
cancer, 4, 52, 55, 71, 72, 74, 89, 91, 128, 138, 144, 145, 180
carbohydrate-restricted diets, 33, 36, 40, 43–44, 48, 81, 85–86, 88–89, 163. *See also individual diets*

Carroll, Peter, 73
CDC (Centers for Disease Control and Prevention), 1, 12, 89
celiac disease, 99
China Study, 38, 40, 71–72, 73
cholesterol, 70, 71, 72, 73
cleanses, 16–22
Cleveland Clinic, 67–68
Clinton, Bill, 57, 63
Clinton, Hillary, 57
Cordain, Loren, 90, 92

D

DeBakey, Michael, 54, 55, 57
de Gaulle, Charles, 149
Devereux, James Raymond, 28–29, 198
diabetes, 4, 12, 52, 54, 57, 64, 71, 72, 91, 97, 138, 145, 162, 166, 172, 180
Dietary Guidelines for Americans, 52, 53
diets
  early, 198–99
  fad, 12–13, 23–34
  instant results and, 15
  lapses during, 12, 121–22
  long-term ineffectiveness of, 13, 30, 181
  See also individual diets
The Drinking Man's Diet, 32–33, 199

E

Eastwood, Clint, 57
Eaton, S. Boyd, 7, 52, 90–93
Edison, Thomas, 27
electrolytes, 21
Esselstyn, Caldwell B., 38, 40, 67–68, 69, 70, 71, 78
exercise, 183, 185–86, 193

F

fad diets, 12–13, 23–34. *See also individual diets*
Fair, William, 73
Farmer, Fannie, 154
Fasano, Alessio, 52
fasting diets, 48
fat-restricted diets, 36, 40, 48, 53–54, 67–68, 69, 70, 78. *See also individual diets*
FDA (Food and Drug Administration), 115
Feinstein, Diane, 63
fiber, importance of, 12, 83, 98, 175
Fischler, Claude, 151, 153, 154, 157
5:2 diet, 48
flavonoids, 144
Fletcher, Anne M., 182, 184
Fletcher, Horace, 26–28, 168, 192, 199
Fletcherism, 26–28
food pyramid, 52

Ford, Henry, 29
Foster, Gary, 114–15, 117–19, 161
Framingham Heart Study, 70, 180
Fraser, Gary, 124, 126, 127–28, 130–31, 161
French approach to eating, 147–58, 194

G

ghrelin, 179
Gingrich, Newt, 63
gluten, 6, 52, 99–100
glycemic index, 52
glycogen, 22
Graham, Letha, 125
Graham, Sylvester, 36–39, 50, 78, 198
Graham-ism, 36–40
Greek diet. *See* Mediterranean diet
Guiliano, Mireille, 156–58, 161, 194–95

H

Hall, Kathryn, 60
Hardinge, Mervyn, 126–27
Harrop, George A., 31, 199
Hartwig, Dallas, 3–4, 6–8, 10–12, 192
Harvey, William, 41, 43
Haseler, Savannah, 9
Hay, William, 29, 199
heart disease, 54–57, 64–65, 67–68, 70, 71, 80, 83, 140–41, 159–60, 165–66
HFCS (high-fructose corn syrup), 169, 170, 171
Hollywood diet, 29, 31, 199
Hu, Frank, 52

I

Ifland, Joan, 165
insulin resistance, 4, 82–83, 171

J

James, Henry, 27
Jenkins, David J. A., 52
Jenny Craig, 48, 112
Jetton, Marge, 124–25
Jobs, Steve, 57
Johns Hopkins University, 25, 31
Jolliffe, Norman, 106–7, 109
Jones, Clancy, 57

K

Kafka, Franz, 27
Kain, Ida Jean, 32
Kane, H. Victor, 33
Kea, 135–36, 138
Kellogg, Ella, 39–40
Kellogg, John Harvey, 31–32, 39–40, 198
Kellogg, Will Keith (W. K.), 40

Kellogg Company, 40
Kerns, Laura, 11–12
keto diets, 42, 44, 87, 95–97
Keys, Ancel, 139–41, 165, 166, 168
Knowles, Beyoncé, 16
Kosinski, Christophe, 96–97
Kraft Heinz Company, 112
Kremezi, Aglaia, 135–36, 138, 139, 142, 144

L

Lee, Dennis, 132–33
Lefer, Mel, 64
The Lemonade Diet. *See* The Master Cleanse
leptin, 167, 171, 179
Levenstein, Harvey, 154
Loma Linda, 123–25, 127, 132–34
Ludwig, David, 13, 161–65
Lustig, Robert, 167, 169, 171–72, 173, 175

M

Malmberg, Carl, 25, 31, 36
The Master Cleanse, 16–22, 23, 24, 25
Mayo Clinic, 180
Mediterranean diet, 52, 68, 136–46
Meilicke, Ethyl, 125
Midler, Bette, 81
milk farms, 32
Minnesota Starvation Study, 140
Mintz, Sidney, 169
Modified Carbohydrate Diet, 81
Moraitis, Costas, 136
Moyer, Melinda, 65–66, 67
Mozaffarian, Dariush, 139

N

Nabel, Elizabeth, 50
National Weight Control Registry, 182, 184–87, 193
Nidetch, Jean, 48, 103, 105–11
nitric oxide, 68
Nordmann, Alain, 88
Nutrisystem, 48, 81, 112
nuts, 128, 130

O

Obama, Barack, 59
Obama, Michelle, 59
obesity, prevalence of, 1, 3, 65, 148
Oldways Preservation Trust, 142
olive oil, 141, 143–44, 197
one-ingredient diets, 31–32
Ornish, Dean, 36, 38, 40, 53–66, 67, 68, 73–78, 127, 136, 161

P

paleo diet, 7–8, 42, 44, 52, 87, 89–95
Pastorino, Briana, 134

Pépin, Jacques, 148–51, 153, 154, 156, 192, 194
Pepino, M. Yanina, 172
Peters, Lulu Hunt, 45–48, 50, 192
praying, 33–34
Presley, Elvis, 32
Preventive Medicine Research Institute, 57, 63
Pritikin, Nathan, 38, 40
processed foods, 163–65, 173
Prudent Diet, 107

R

recipes, 191–92
refined carbohydrates, 163–65, 195
Rich, Irene, 32
Rockefeller, John D., 27
Rozin, Paul, 154, 156, 157

S

Sabaté, Joan, 52
Sacks, Frank, 48
Salisbury, James Henry, 28, 198
Salisbury System of Weight Reduction, 28, 198
Sanfilippo, Diane, 90
Satchidananda, Swami, 62
saturated fat, 52, 84, 92, 140–41, 143, 165, 168
Sawyer, Jennifer, 134
Scarsdale Diet, 42, 43–44, 46
Seinfeld, Jerry, 193
Seven Countries Study, 140
Seventh-Day Adventists, 38, 39, 40, 125–34, 193
Shedd, Charlie W., 33
sleep, 178–79
Sleeping Beauty diet, 32
Smith, Mark, 99–100
South Beach Diet, 12, 42, 44, 79–85, 97–100, 192
Spencer-Hwang, Rhonda, 125
Stampfer, Meir, 52
starvation response, 164
Stefansson, Vilhjalmur, 165
Steffen, Lyn, 65
Sterne, Laurence, 47
Stevens, Molly, 99–100
sugar, 163, 165–75
sweeteners, artificial, 172–73
Swithers, Susan, 172

T

Tate, Deborah, 119
Taubes, Gary, 64–65
Thomas, J. Graham, 181–82, 184–87
time-restricted diets, 48
Trichopoulou, Antonia, 52, 141–44, 146, 161
Twain's Brewpub and Billiards, 9–10
two-ingredient diets, 31

U
United Fruit Company, 31
Urban, Melissa, 3–4, 6–8, 10–12, 192
USDA (US Department of Agriculture), 10

V
Vogel, Leanne, 96

W
Wareham, Ellsworth, 125
Warinner, Christina, 93
weight loss
  exercise and, 183, 185–86
  health benefits of, 2, 185
  individualized approach to, 184–85, 190–97
  successful long-term, 181–82, 184–87, 191
weight management industry, size of, 12–13
Weight Watchers, 47, 48, 101, 105, 109–13, 192. *See also* WW International
Western Health Reform Institute, 39, 198
White, Ellen, 39, 125–26, 127, 198
The Whole30, 3–14, 23, 24, 25, 42, 44, 112, 193
Whole Foods Market, 3
Willett, Walter, 53, 132
wine, 144, 146, 180
Winfrey, Oprah, 102
Winter, Christopher, 179
Wolf, Robb, 90
Wood, Minnie, 125
WW International, 47, 48, 101–5, 110, 111–22, 165

Y
Yudkin, John, 165–66, 168, 171, 175

Z
Zheng, Yaguang, 12
The Zone, 12, 42, 44
Zuk, Marlene, 94

Also by Barry Estabrook

Tomatoland: How Modern Industrial Agriculture Destroyed Our Most Alluring Fruit

Pig Tales: An Omnivore's Quest for Sustainable Meat

Published in the United States by Lorena Jones Books, an imprint of Random House, a division of Penguin Random House LLC, New York.
www.tenspeed.com

Lorena Jones Books and the Lorena Jones Books colophon are trademarks of Penguin Random House, LLC.

Library of Congress Cataloging-in-Publication Data on file with publisher.

Hardcover ISBN: 978-0-399-58027-7
Ebook ISBN: 978-0-399-58028-4

Printed in the United States of America

Designer: Isabelle Gioffredi
Production designer: Mari Gill
Production manager: Dan Myers
Copyeditor: Deborah Kops
Proofreader: Andrea Chesman
Indexer: Ken DellaPenta

Cover image by Ilyashenko Oleksiy/Shutterstock.com
Icons on the cover and pages 5, 17, 38, 42, 46, 49, 58, 69, 87, 110, 116, 129, 137, 145, 152, 155, 167, 170, 183, and 197 by Kakosha/Shutterstock.com

10 9 8 7 6 5 4 3 2 1

First Edition